The Power of Positive Coloring

Creating Digital Downtime for Self-Discovery

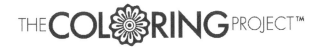

Andrea Reyna Kohler

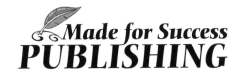
Made for Success
PUBLISHING

INTRODUCTION

The Power of Positive Coloring is designed to blend the benefits of coloring and the work of self-discovery. In today's busy world, it's challenging to find time to slow down and carve out intentional space for ourselves. Coloring is a wonderful tool for a mindfulness practice and supports this type of focus. Its benefits include:

Calm: Slow down. Focus on one thing. Relax your body by engaging your creative, logical and kinesthetic brain all at the same time.

Create: Access your own creativity and self-expression with a structure that's a little less scary than a blank page and an instruction to draw.

Get Clear: Shift your focus from your "to do" list to coloring, creativity, to the "doing" of art. Clear your thoughts to create the thinking space for new ideas to surface.

Get Conscious: Coloring can serve as an active meditation. Choose an intention, an idea, a concept a thought or a mantra to focus on while you color.

Connect: Use the DigitalDowntime™ to connect with yourself or, if you're coloring in a group, deepen the discussion, let the conversation flow, and allow connections to be made.

Each illustration features a word or a quote to focus on while you color. On the opposite page, you'll find a quote aligned with the illustration's message, and a mindfulness activity with before and after sections designed to help you focus your time spent coloring. The **While You Color** activities focus on deepening awareness and exploring intentions, the **Take a Moment** activities help you put your new awareness into action.

You will also find a quote aligned with the word or phrase in the illustration – just one more way to take your coloring deeper, as a tool for focus and mindfulness practice.

HOW TO USE THIS BOOK

Before you color, take a moment to create your environment. Find a place to sit, the right light, turn on some music and settle in.

Take another moment to focus yourself, clear your mind and set the intention for your coloring session. Take a few deep breaths, inhaling deeply and exhaling completely. Feel your feet connected to the floor, feel your body start to relax even before you begin.

Choose an illustration. Flip through the pages and find an illustration (the word or phrase) that resonates with you. Or, you can go page by page, in order. Whatever feels right to you. Read the mindfulness activity on the opposite page and get your COLORING on!

When you're finished, read through the **Take a Moment** section and answer the simple questions. These are designed to help you take your journey of self-discovery and moments of mindfulness just a little bit further.

We all are capable of greatness. It's within us. It's in our DNA. We all have an inner dialogue – a story we tell ourselves about what we are capable of – what is possible for us. Our stories create our expectations, our reality and our limits.

What story do you tell yourself? What untapped capability is on the other side of your story? Focus on creating a story that empowers you. When you envision something, you create the ability to achieve it.

While you color, shake off those doubts and fears and ponder how truly capable you really are.

- *What do you want to create? What are things that you know, deep down, that you are capable of doing?*

- *What things have you already accomplished? How did you know you could do it? What did you focus on?*

- *Who are the people who help you remember your power and strength.*

Take a moment to go deeper. Answer the questions below and record any musings, epiphanies or thoughts you want to remember.

1. Think about something that you are focused on accomplishing. What is one thing that you will do this week to work towards your goal?

_____

_____

2. What is one thing that you accomplished in the past that you didn't think you could do?

_____

_____

"If we did all the things we are capable of, we would literally astound ourselves."

~Thomas Edison

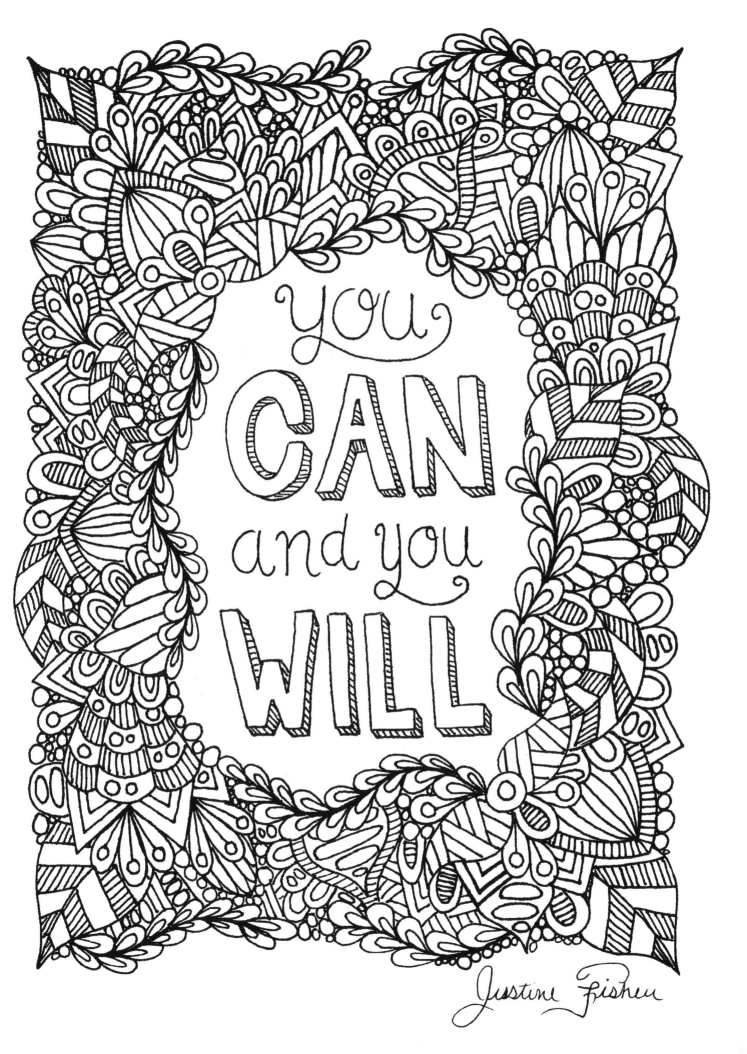

Choices. We make dozens of them every day – some little, some big, some are intentional and some come from our automatic response patterns.

One of the most important choices we get to make is who we are.

We have a choice. We get to choose. We get to choose what we cultivate within ourselves. We get to decide who we are, what we focus on, and how we show up in life.

At every moment of every day, we have a choice.

As you color, ponder who you chose to be. Are you happy with who you are? Are there any adjustments you want to make? If there aren't any, that's simply another choice you get to make.

- *What are your favorite parts of yourself? How do you cultivate them?*
- *How do you describe yourself? I'm a _____ kind of person, I'm not a _____ kind of person.*
- *What are the parts of yourself that you have intentionally developed? If so, what are they and why did you choose them?*

Take a moment to go deeper. Answer the questions below and record any musings, epiphanies, or thoughts you want to remember.

1. Write down 5 words that describe you.

_____

_____

2. What is a quality about yourself that you intentionally choose to cultivate? What is one thing you can do this week to cultivate it?

_____

_____

"Who do you want to be today? Who do you want to be?"

~ Danny Elfman, Oingo Boingo

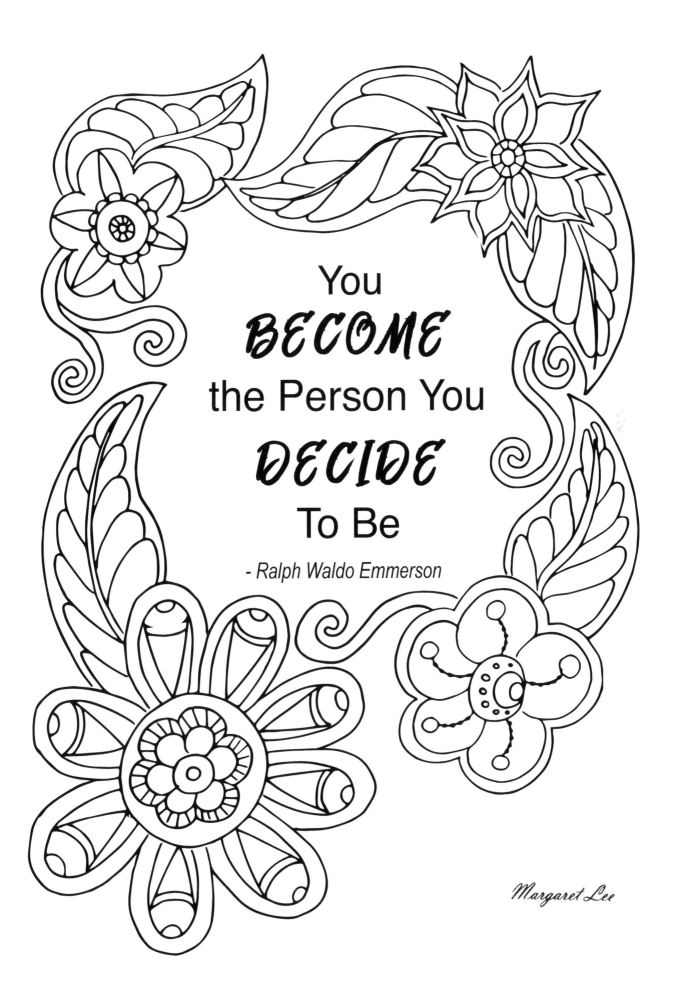

You
BECOME
the Person You
DECIDE
To Be

- Ralph Waldo Emmerson

Margaret Lee

"Careful the words you say, children will listen." ~ Stephen Sondheim

Words are powerful. We listen to every word we say – those spoken out loud and those whispered quietly to ourselves.

Words form thoughts. Thoughts create our personal story and how we think about ourselves. Thoughts also create action – before we do anything, we have to think of it.

Thoughts create beliefs. When we believe something, we gravitate towards it, we look for evidence to reinforce it. We attract things that resonate with our beliefs, and we create actions and habits that align with them.

Thoughts, when repeated, create habits. Habits begin to create character.

Careful the things you say – you are listening, you are thinking, you are beginning to believe.

While you color, take this opportunity to get to know and explore your inner dialogue.

- *Notice your internal dialogue. What does it say to you?*

- *Is your internal dialogue positive or negative? What does it tell you about your abilities?*

- *Is the story you're telling yourself the one you want to create? Are there any changes you want to make to your inner dialogue?*

Take a moment to go deeper. Answer the questions below and record any musings, epiphanies, or thoughts you want to remember.

1. Is there anything about your inner dialogue you want to change? If yes, write down what you would like to change.

_____

_____

2. What is one action you can take this week to be intentional about your inner dialogue?

_____

_____

"Your beliefs become your thoughts,
Your thoughts become your words,
Your words become your actions,
Your actions become your habits,
Your habits become your values,
Your values become your destiny."
~ Mahatma Gandhi

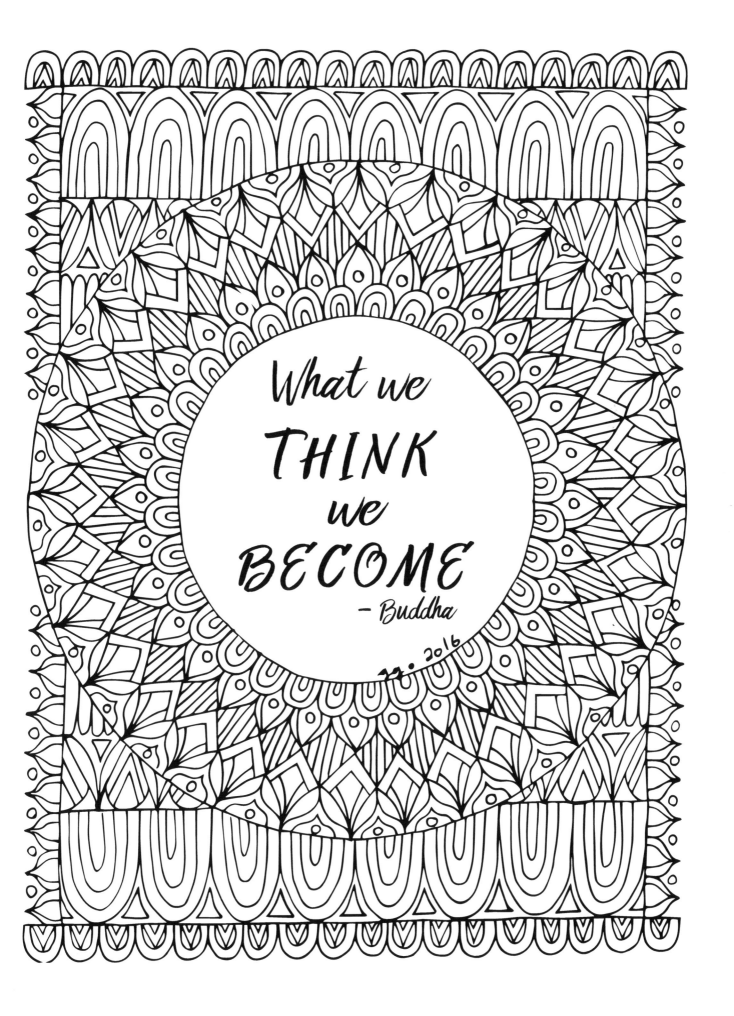

Everyday we talk, we type, we text, we check Facebook, we click 'like' on things as we scroll, we "connect." However, in this world of constant connection, it can be very easy to NOT feel connected.

Feeling connected (to others AND to ourselves) is good for us – mentally, physically, emotionally, creatively, etc. Feeling connected contributes to us feeling worthy and loveable. In fact, research has shown that the feeling of connection not only helps us feel good – but helps us do good. Finding time to connect with your own inner compass and with others is necessary.

While you color, put those digital distractions aside and spend a few moments pondering what connection feels like.

- *When was the last time you felt really connected? What did it feel like?*
- *What things do you do to feel connected? What are your go to connection activities?*
- *What is your favorite way to connect... to yourself or to others?*

Take a moment to go deeper. Answer the questions below and record any musings, epiphanies, or thoughts you want to remember.

1. Do you feel connected to your inner compass? How is your inner compass feeling?

_____

_____

2. What are two things you can do this week to feel more connected?

_____

_____

"We do not find the meaning of life by ourselves alone - we find it with another."

~ Thomas Merton

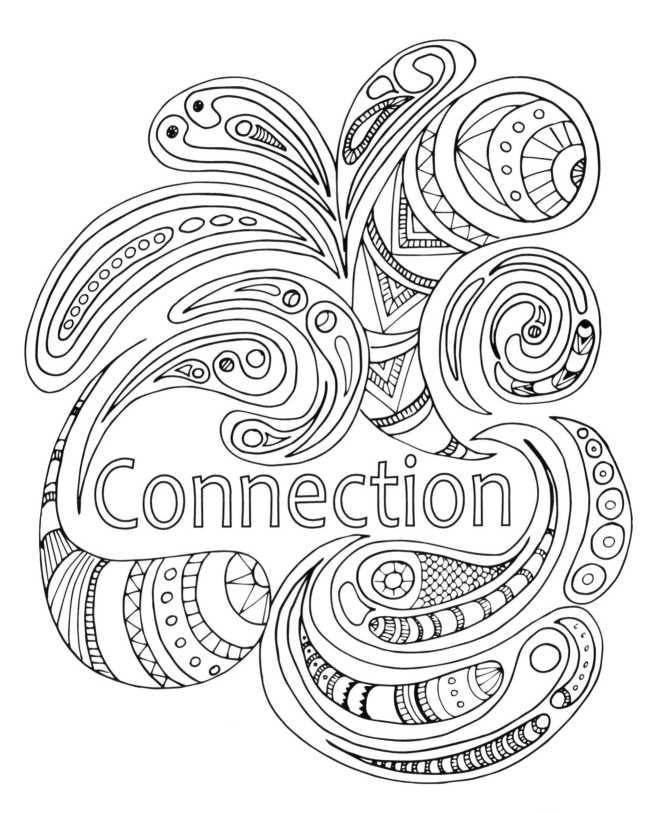

Margaret Lee

Self-Care. Your car requires fuel. Your phone needs its battery. Your body needs food. Your soul and spirit also need love.

It's easy to prioritize others' needs above your own, to take care of yourself after you've attended to everyone else.

Self love is not selfish. Loving yourself first means doing what you need to do to fulfill yourself, so that you have more love to share.

Self-care is unique, and what recharges you is specific to you. Is it getting enough sleep? Getting enough exercise? Is it more social time with friends, or less? Sometimes self-care means buckling down and pulling an all-nighter when a project is due. Sometimes it means taking a break, taking a walk, or watching your favorite 'brain candy' television show. Whatever it looks like for you, whatever you know that you need, self-care is a way to honor yourself.

While you color, check in with yourself about what self-care looks like for you.

- *What are the things you do that help you rejuvenate and refuel?*
- *When you need to 'reboot,' where do you go? Who do you call?*

Take a moment to go deeper. Answer the questions below and record any musings, epiphanies, or thoughts you want to remember.

1. What is your go to self-care routine?

_____

_____

2. What will you do this week for self-care? How will you love yourself first this week?

_____

_____

"Love yourself first and everything else falls into line. You really have to love yourself to get anything done in this world."

~ Lucille Ball

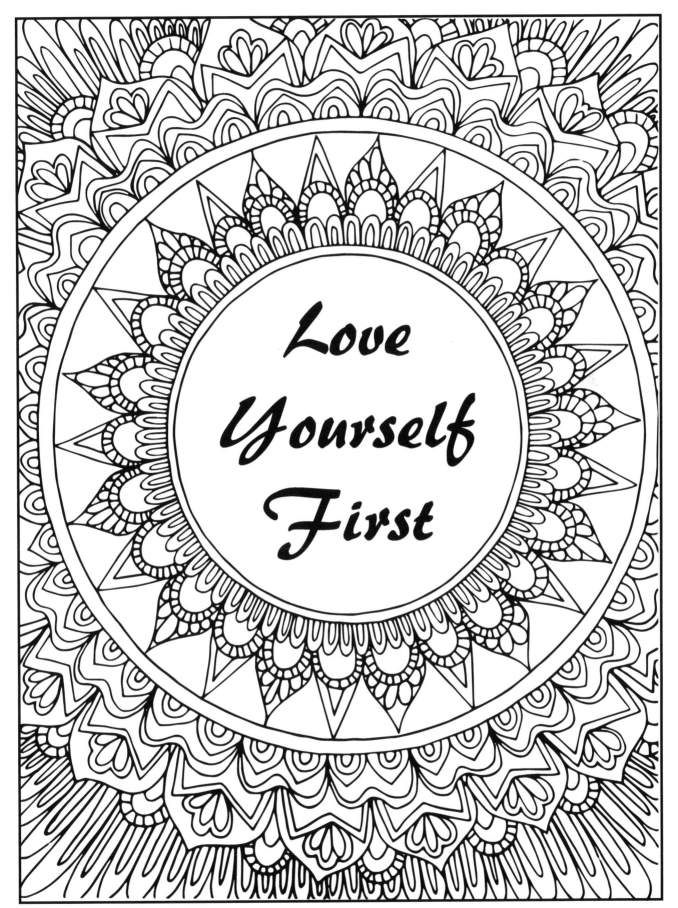

Love Yourself First

Shhhhh. Can you hear it? It's your intuition, instinct, inner compass or – simply – your gut.

Whatever you call it, it's that voice inside us, the one that steers us towards what we want and away from the things we don't.

It's that feeling when you know something is right and you should keep going.

It's that shadow of doubt that shows up when something just doesn't sit quite right.

Sometimes it speaks loudly and sometimes it's only a soft whisper. Sometimes it can be hard to hear over the other, louder voices telling you what they think you should do.

You can feel it. You know it's there. Trust it.

While you color, check in with your inner voice and spend some time getting to know it.

- *How does your inner voice speak to you? What does it sound like? What does it feel like?*
- *What things do you do that help you tune into your inner voice?*
- *What are some examples of when you have listened to your inner voice?*

Take a moment to go deeper. Answer the questions below and record any musings, epiphanies, or thoughts you want to remember.

1. What is an example of a time that you listened to your inner voice, your intuition, your gut?

_____

_____

2. What one action you can take this week to tune into your inner voice?

_____

_____

"Don't let the noise of others' opinions drown out your own inner voice."

~ Steve Jobs
[Stanford University commencement speech, 2005]

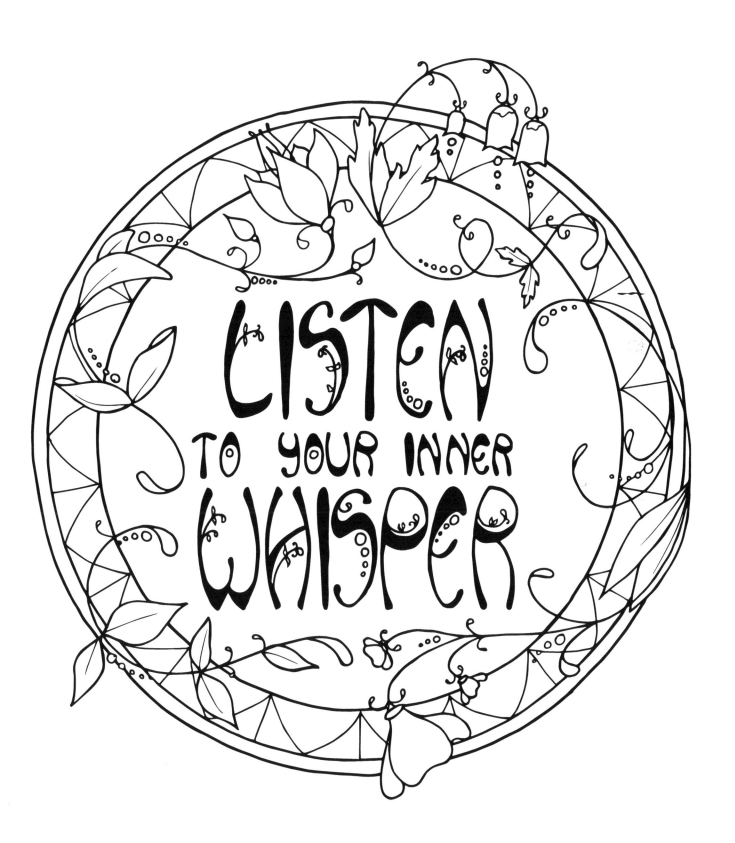

Fear is a 4-letter word. It tells us that change, or anything outside our comfort zone, is scary. It says things like "what if." It shows up as "if only" and "when I'm ready," helping us believe that if we just wait, it will be easier or less scary.

You know those dreams you have, those things that you want to do? They're possible. They're just hanging out, over there, on the other side of fear.

Will you be nervous? Yes. Will you do it perfectly the first time? Probably not.

If you can't dive into your dream yet – dip your toe in, baby step, or just look in the general direction of your dream. You have the power to ignite your dreams.

While you color, check in with your dreams and then with your comfort zone, get to know it, say hello.

- *Where is the edge of your comfort zone and what does it feel like?*
- *What are your "what ifs" and "if onlys?" What would be possible if they disappeared?*

Take a moment to go deeper. Answer the questions below and record any musings, epiphanies, or thoughts you want to remember.

1. What is one thing that used to be out of your comfort zone that is not anymore?

_____

_____

2. What is one action you can take to grow your comfort zone this week?

_____

*"There is freedom waiting for you,
On the breezes of the sky,
And you ask "What if I fall?"
Oh but my darling,
What if you fly?"*

~Erin Hanson

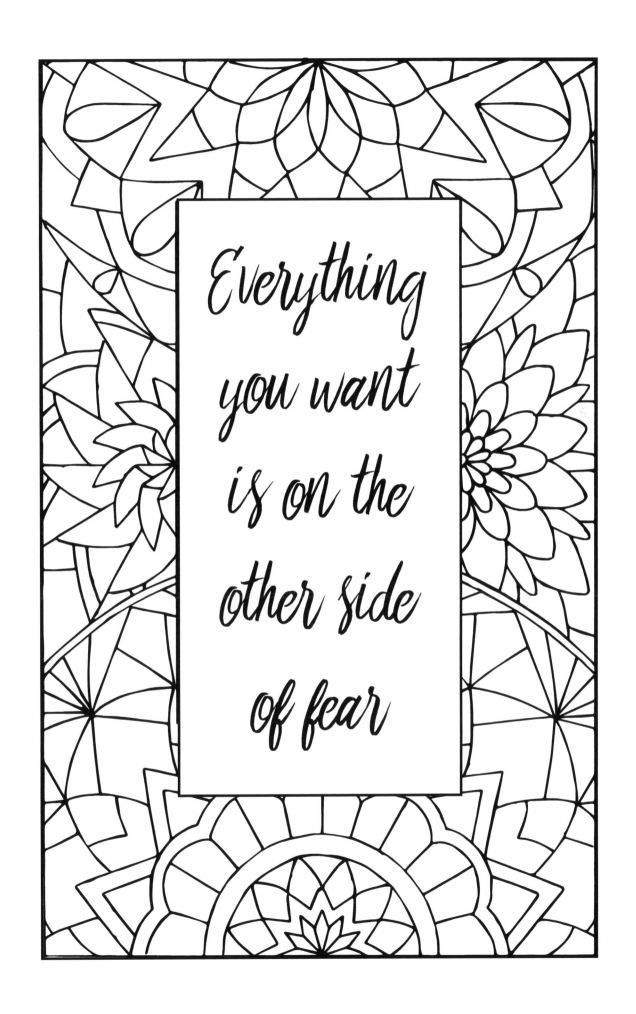

Everything you want is on the other side of fear

What does freedom mean to you? Freedom can mean many things. It can be linked to independence, liberty, an absence of restrictions. It may mean the ability to exercise one's rights, powers, or desires. It may mean the freedom of speech, of conscience, or of movement. It might mean choosing what books you read, when you want to go to bed, or who you get to hang out with.

Freedom can also mean the ability to choose what we do with information, to choose what stories we create for ourselves. We get to interpret our life, to create our future, to change our minds, to learn from our mistakes. Freedom can mean choosing what we believe.

As you color, take a few minutes to ponder what freedom means to you?

- *What does freedom feel like for you? What does it look like? What does it sound like?*

- *Is feeling free important to you? Why?*

- *When and where do you feel the most free?*

Take a moment to go deeper. Answer the questions below and record any musings, epiphanies, or thoughts you want to remember.

1. What are three things that freedom means to you?

_____

_____

2. What actions will you take this week to feel free?

_____

_____

*"I know but one freedom and that is
the freedom of the mind."*

~Antoine de Saint-Exuper

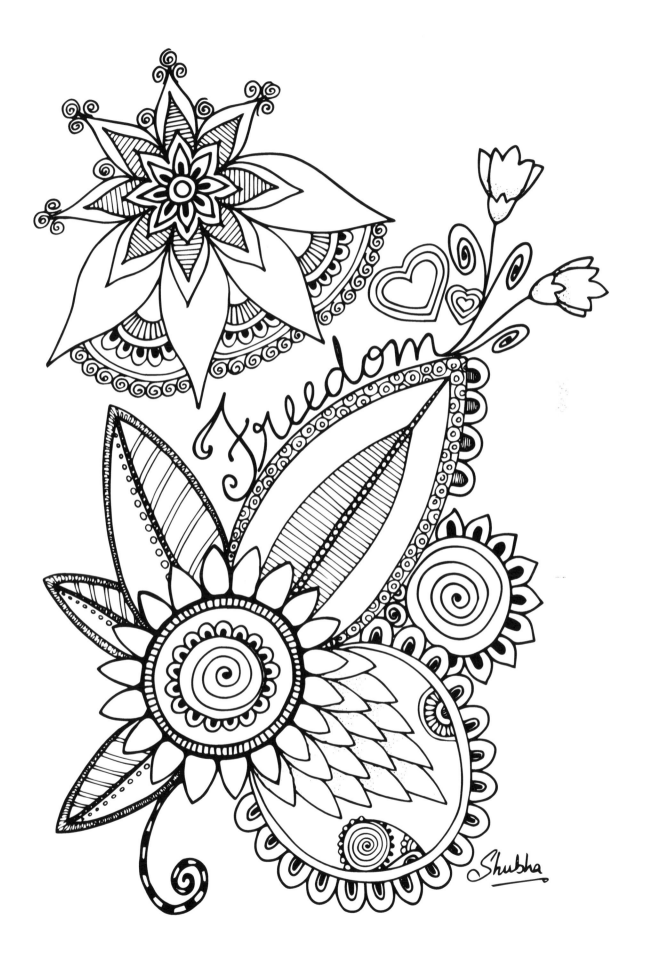

Intention is the starting point to everything. It is the creative power behind our thoughts, our beliefs, and our actions.

Our intentions are like seeds that, after being planted, grow. And, just as with a seed, intention is watered with our thoughts and actions. What grows is the result of the seed we planted. Our reality is the result of the intention we hold and the thoughts and actions we take.

Intentions can be physical, social, emotional, financial, etc.

Intentions can be general or they can be very specific.

Intentions can be focused on the bigger picture or on daily needs.

What are your intentions manifesting?

While you color, connect to your intentions and what you want to manifest in life.

- *What does it feel like to be intentional?*
- *What are your intentions in your personal life? Professional life?*
- *What changes when you are being intentional?*

Take a moment to go deeper. Answer the questions below and record any musings, epiphanies, or thoughts you want to remember.

1. What is one thing that you have manifested through intentions in the past?

_____

_____

2. Think of one intention you have. Write it down. Now, think about everything surrounding that intention, the why, the what, the when, where and how. Write that down too.

_____

_____

"You are what your deepest desire is. As your desire is, so is your intention. As your intention is, so is your will. As your will is, so is your deed. As your deed is, so is your destiny."

~ The Upanishads

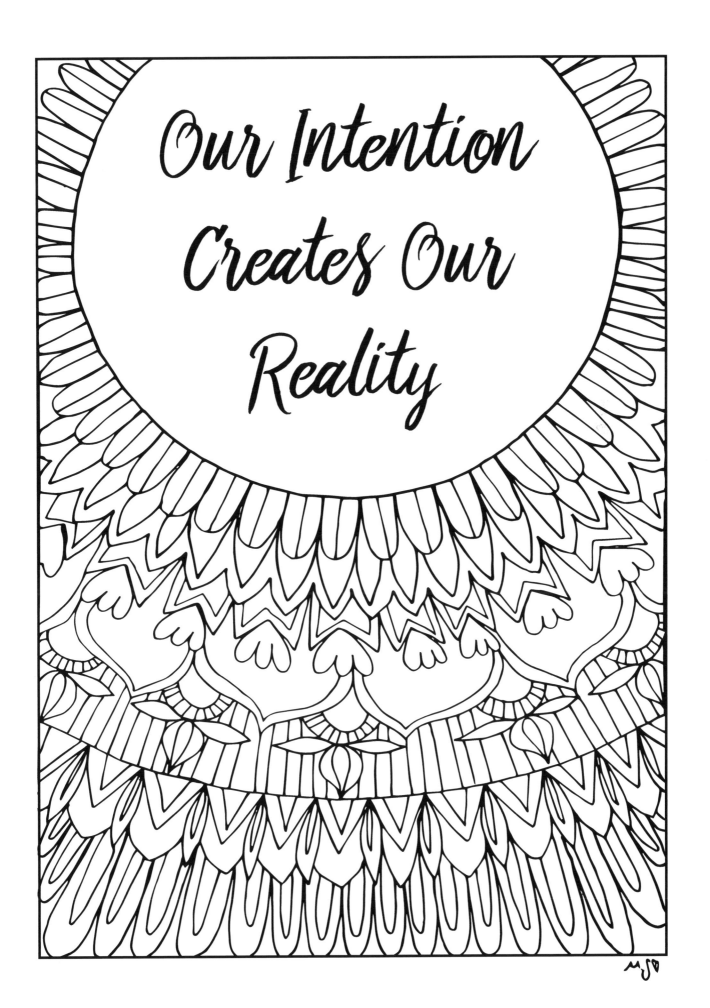

"Tell me what you want, what you really, really want." ~ The Spice Girls

But, all joking and the Spice Girls aside, PURPOSE provides FOCUS. Period.

Knowing your WHY helps you create a life that you love. Knowing your WHY helps you stay committed. When life throws you its curve balls, knowing your WHY helps you find courage and provides power and energy resources to take the risks needed and do the things you are passionate about.

While you color, fine tune your inner compass so that it can point to the thing(s) that are at your 'true North.' Try focusing on the questions below:

- *What makes you feel alive? What gets you out of bed in the morning?*

- *What is your 'siren' – that thing that you are so passionate about that it just keeps calling to you?*

- *What would YOU say is your purpose?*

Take a moment to go deeper. Answer the questions below and record any musings, epiphanies, or thoughts you want to remember.

1. What would you say your purpose is? Remember, there's no right or wrong – your purpose is what you say it is, and that you can have more than one purpose.

_____

_____

2. What will you do this week to tune your inner compass?

_____

_____

"He who has a WHY can endure any HOW."
~ Frederick Nietzche

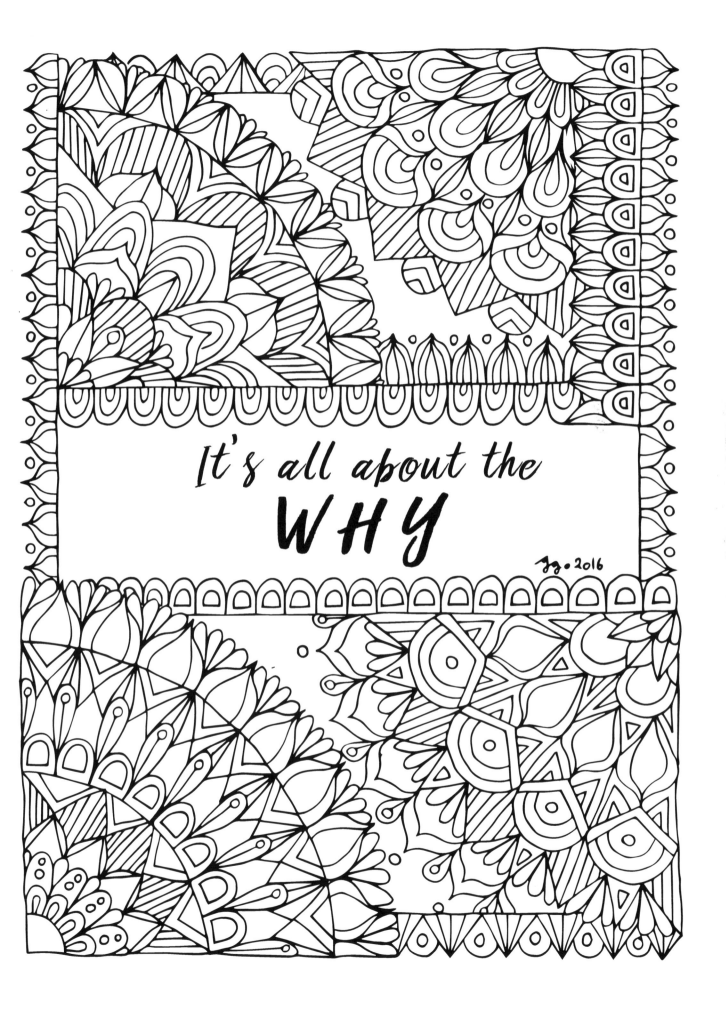

Just as you are. Because you are. Because you exist. You are enough.

There is no final authority on "enough," no Wizard behind the green curtain, no dictionary definition of what you need to be to be "enough."

You are as unique as the specific combination of mind blowing biology that brought you into existence. There is no one else that will ever be as good at being you, than you!

You have nothing to prove, no one to live up to. The path is yours to create.

You are beyond comparison. You, alone, are enough.

While coloring, begin to ponder the sheer awesomeness that is all that you are. Begin to explore all that you're capable of and all the dreams that you have.

- *What are your favorite, unique qualities about yourself?*
- *What about you are you proud of?*
- *What are your strengths?*
- *What can you do that no one else can?*

Take a moment to go deeper. Answer the questions below and record any musings, epiphanies, or thoughts you want to remember.

1. What is something about that you wouldn't change, no matter what?

_____

_____

2. What is one thing you know about yourself to be true?

_____

_____

"The easiest thing to be in the world is you. The most difficult thing to be is what other people want you to be."

~ Leo Buscaglia

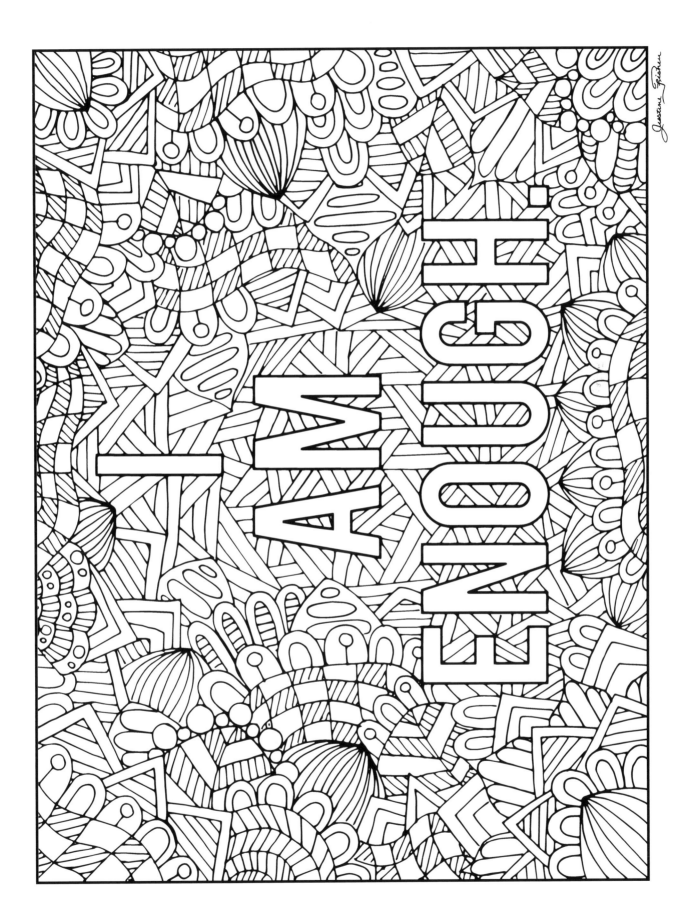

The world would shift magnificently if each person on the planet were able to see the greatness that resides within themselves.

We hold ourselves back, afraid that who we are is not what the world wants. We look for approval, for someone to counter the inner belief that somehow we are less than worthy.

You are a gift. You are the only one born with your unique set of talents. You do not need approval to you be you. You do not need to please anyone but yourself. Get to know all of the nooks and crannies of your personality.

Embrace ALL that you are.

While you color, take this time to get to know all of your qualities and explore all that you are.

- *What are the traits that you possess that are uniquely you? Are you Smart, Funny, Creative, Introspective, Thoughtful, etc.?*

- *What roles do you play in life? Are you a sibling, a parent, a child, a coworker, a teacher, etc.?*

- *What do you value? What's important to you?*

- *What would it feel like to embrace all that you are, completely?*

Take a moment to go deeper. Answer the questions below and record any musings, epiphanies, or thoughts you want to remember.

1. What are two of your favorite traits? Why?

_____

_____

2. What is one of the roles that you play? What do you appreciate about it?

_____

_____

"The hardest challenge is to be yourself in a world where everyone is trying to make you be somebody else."

~ E. E. Cummings

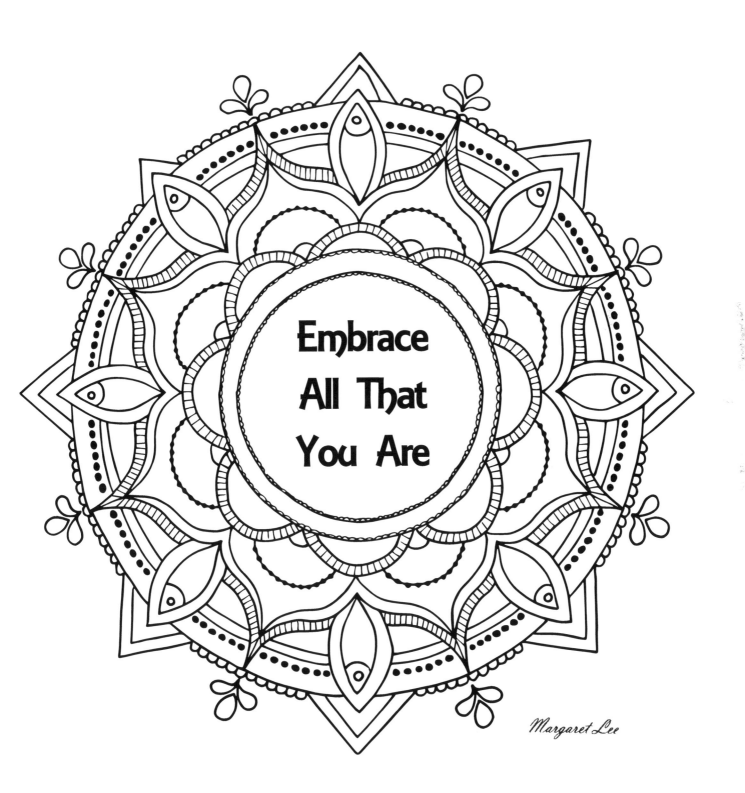

Embrace
All That
You Are

Margaret Lee

Passion. Heat. Fire. Desire.

Our passion make us feel alive. It's that strong emotion you have inside that drives you and keeps you fueled through the day. It's what you fight for. Passion is what you do even when you don't have to.

Passion allows us to see potential, to focus, to trust ourselves, to take risks, and to overcome obstacles.

Like rocket fuel, passion is your hobby, amplified, all-out, taken to the next level. Passion is that force that has you go "Full Nerd" and not care one bit. You can't tone it down. You can't switch it off.

While you color, think about what you are passionate about – is it singing? Cooking? Gardening? Disassembling gadgets? Or is it reading, dancing, fashion, etc.?

- *What has you staying up through all hours of the night to finish?*
- *What is it that you can't NOT do?*

Take a moment to go deeper. Answer the questions below and record any musings, epiphanies, or thoughts you want to remember.

1. What are the passions that you know you have?

_____

_____

2. What is something that makes you go "Full Nerd?"

_____

_____

*"Passion is one great force that unleashes creativity,
because if you're passionate about something, then
you're more willing to take risks."*

~ Yo-Yo Ma

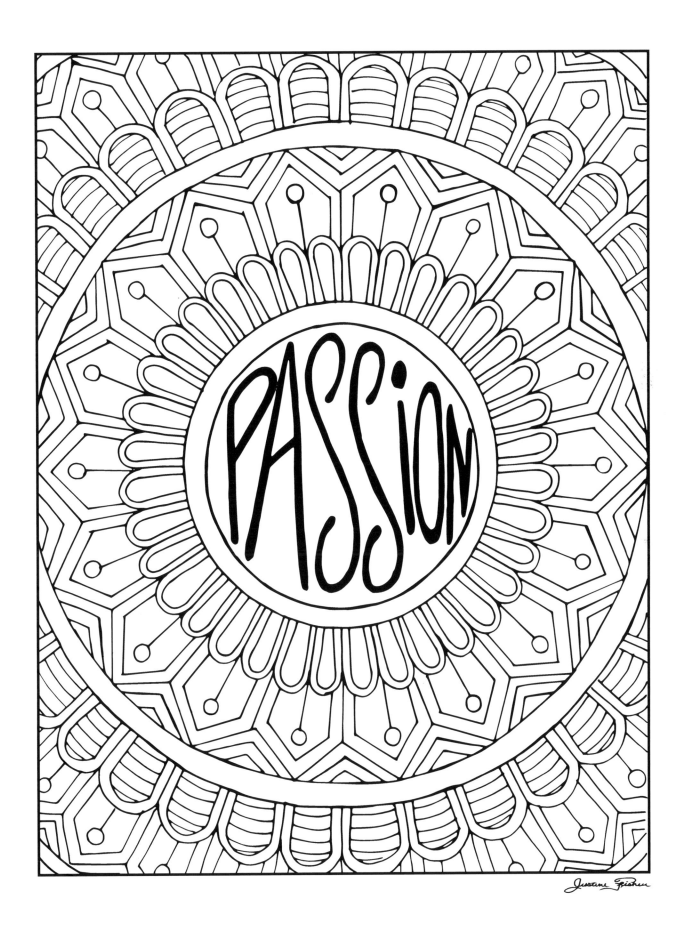

Have you ever met that person that just embodies joy – they love their life, they are always having a good time, they always seem to have a smile on their face? These people are magnetic – you just want to be around them.

Joy is unique in the way it is felt. Joy is also unique in the way it is generated. Joy can come from big things or little things – A great evening out with friends, seeing your favorite musician in concert, a clean house, bedtime for the 9 year old, or just listening to your favorite song while you're stuck in traffic.

Becoming aware of where joy comes from, for you, gives you the power to amplify it. The more YOU know where YOUR joy comes from, the more joy you create and the more joy you attract.

While you color, explore what joy feels like for you and where you find it.

- *What do you do to feel joy? Where do you go? What do you listen to?*
- *When was the last time you felt joy?*
- *Who are some of the people you know who are "joy magnets?"*

Take a moment to go deeper. Answer the questions below and record any musings, epiphanies, or thoughts you want to remember.

1. What are two things that you do to feel joy?

_____

_____

2. What is one thing you can do this week that will remind you to be joyful?

_____

_____

"Joy is the most magnetic force in the Universe."
~ Danielle LaPorte

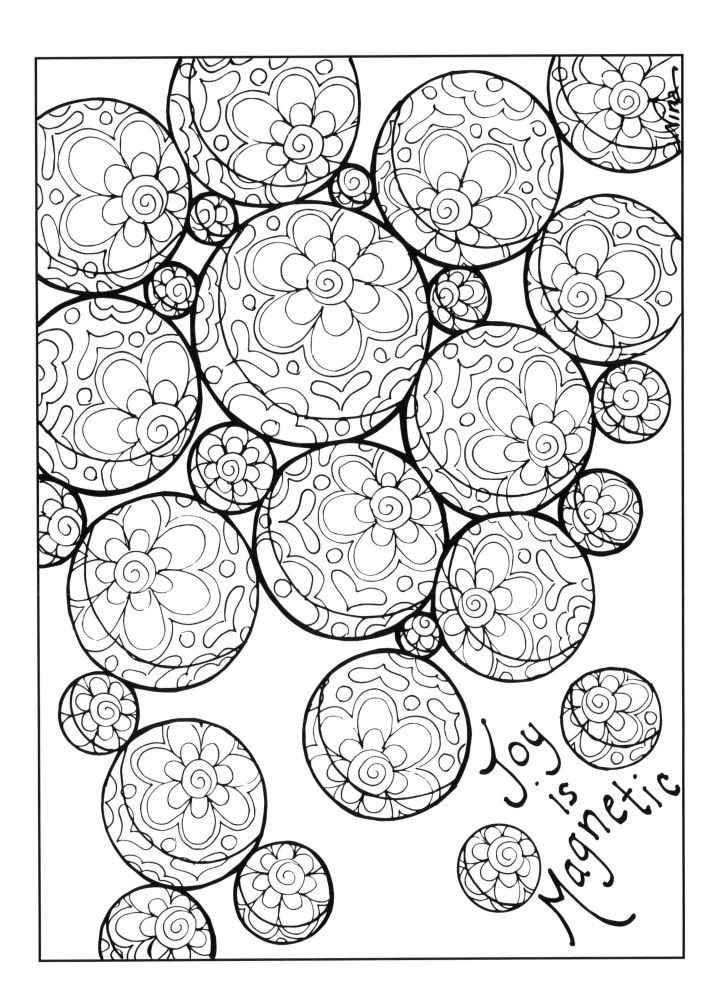

Joy is Magnetic

The definition of 'Love' in the dictionary tells you something like this: "an intense feeling of deep affection." Thanks for the simple explanation of what can be the most complex feeling in the world.

However, LOVE is simple. It is free. It can't be bought or sold. It cannot be traded. It has no territory or borders. It's a noun. It's a verb, adverb and adjective. Love, it's bigger than you, bigger than me, bigger than all of us. Love generates love.

While you color, ponder your feelings surrounding love, what it means for you personally, and how it shows up in your life. This is an invitation to intentionally step into your heart, see what's there, and how much love you can generate.

- *What does love feel like for you?*
- *What do you feel love for in your life?*
- *Who are the people in your life that make you experience love?*
- *What things do you do to feel love?*

Take a moment to go deeper. Answer the questions below and then record any musings, epiphanies, or thoughts you want to remember.

1. Make a list of the ways that you can generate love.

_____

_____

2. What is one thing that you can do to generate love for yourself today?

_____

_____

"Open your heart. ... In your heart is all the love you need. Your heart can create any amount of love, not just for yourself, but for the whole world."
~ Don Miguel Ruiz

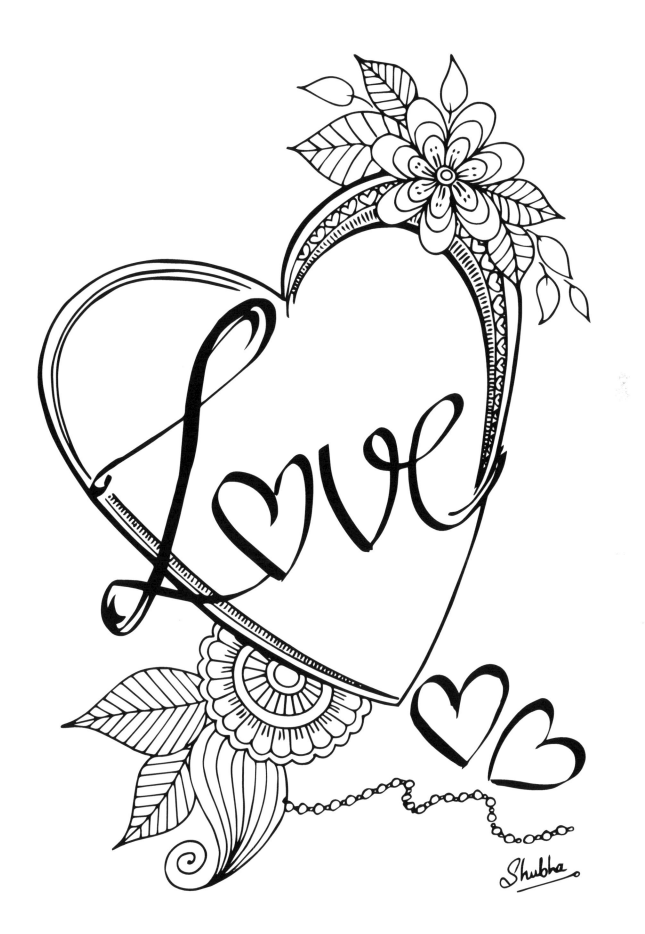

You are the author, engineer, choreographer, and pilot of your life.

The story we live is created from what we believe about our abilities, duties, possibilities, what our bodies look like, how smart we can be, etc. These beliefs impact our identity, our sense of self. They create the story we tell ourselves about who we are.

Beliefs can be positive – *I'm good at this, I can try anything, etc.*

But often, beliefs can be limiting – I'm just not good with money, I can't pursue that dream, I don't know where to start, I'm just not creative, etc.

By exploring what you believe and why you believe it, you give yourself power. You are the writer of this story and YOU can change the narrative. What story do you want to create?

While you color, check in with your own personal story and get familiar with it. What is your personal story telling you?

- *Listen closely. What is your inner critic telling you? How would your life change if you decided to rewrite your inner critic's script?*

- *As the author of your personal story, what changes would you make? What would you make possible?*

Take a moment to go deeper. Answer the questions below and record any musings, epiphanies, or thoughts you want to remember.

1. What is one change to your personal story that you want to make?

_____

_____

2. What is one action you can do this week to make that change?

_____

_____

"Whether you think you can, or whether you think you can't, you are probably right."

~ Henry Ford

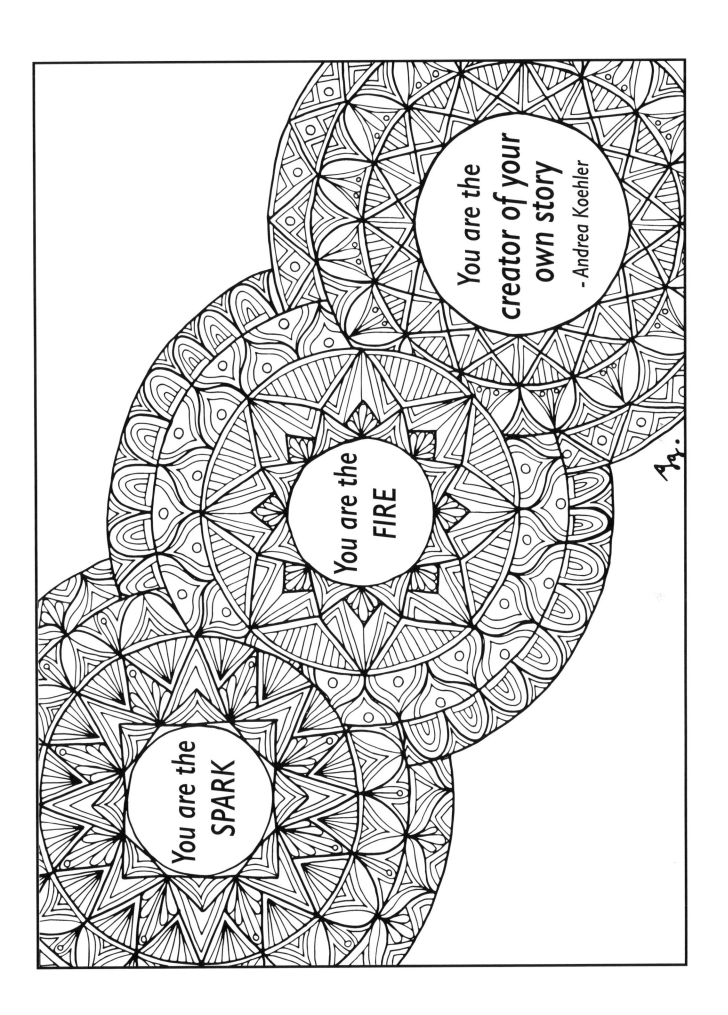

Who am I? A question we have all asked ourselves.

Answers range from our given names to our careers, from the roles we play to our hobbies, from the countries or cultures we come from to what we're passionate about, and from our personalities to our intelligence and characteristics.

I am... a reader, thinker, creator, dancer, pilot, coder, etc.
I am... a sibling, parent, grandchild, member, contributor, etc.
I am... compassionate, kind, loving, joyous, etc.

When you answer this question, you declare how you see yourself and what you believe to be true about you. You declare how you see yourself, through your filters, through your thoughts and your opinions. You construct your foundation. With foundation comes direction. With direction comes purpose.

You are in charge of the definition of you... and no one else.

While you color, connect with who you are – finish the sentence "I am... " with ALL that you are.

- *What roles, activities and personality traits describe you?*

- *What qualities do you display when you are doing things that are important to you?*

Take a moment to go deeper. Answer the questions below and record any musings, epiphanies, or thoughts you want to remember.

1. Finish the sentence "I am..." with at least three examples.

_____

_____

2. What is one activity that you do that helps you feel authentically you?

_____

_____

"The privilege of a lifetime is being who you are."
~ Joseph Campbell

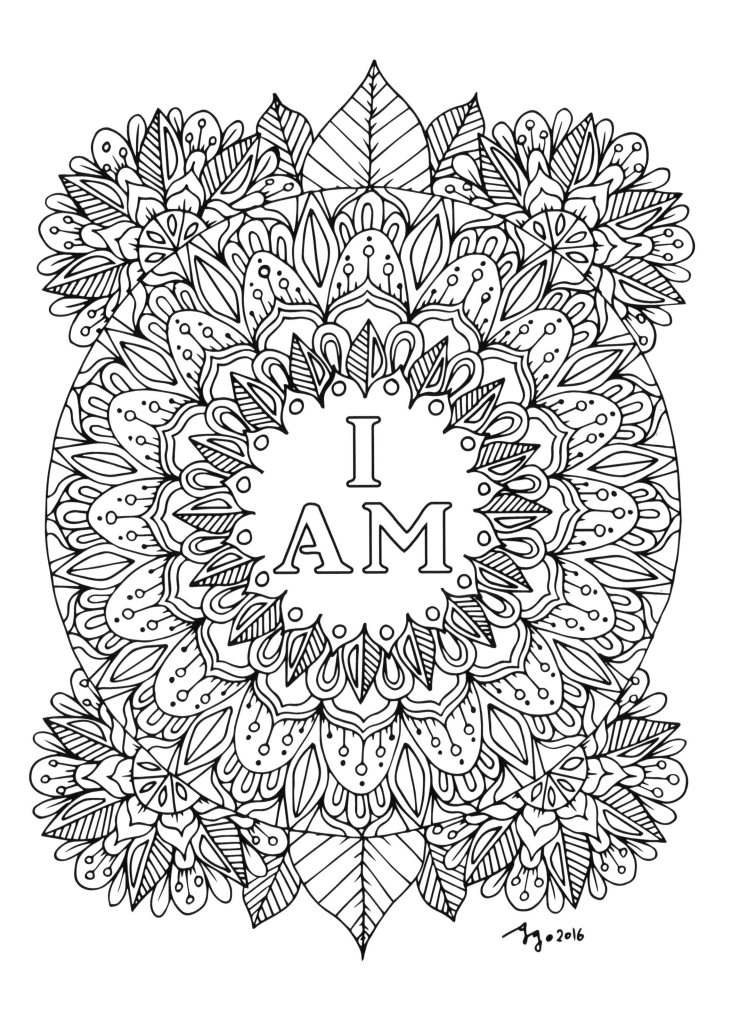

We would all like a magic wand, right? Often times we look outside ourselves for the answers – to that quote, that person, that book that knows "better" than we do. We wait for the timing to be just right. We wait for a magician to wave their magic wand and make all the stars align.

That magical wand you seek? It resides within you.

You. Your MAGIC. Your joy. You are powerful. You are capable. The Magic is already inside.

While you color, imagine that you have been given a magic wand.

- *If there are no limits, what would you change or create? What dream would your magic wand make possible?*

- *Where do you find YOUR magic? With friends? A certain place?*

- *What would you change or create in the following areas:*

  - *At home*

  - *At work*

  - *In relationships (personal and professional)*

  - *Your health*

  - *Your hobbies*

Take a moment to go deeper. Answer the questions below and record any musings, epiphanies, or thoughts you want to remember.

1. What things do you want your MAGIC to change?

_____

_____

2. What is one thing that you will bring your MAGIC to this week?

_____

_____

"Magic is believing in yourself, if you can do that,
you can make anything happen."
~ Johann Wolfgang Von Goethe

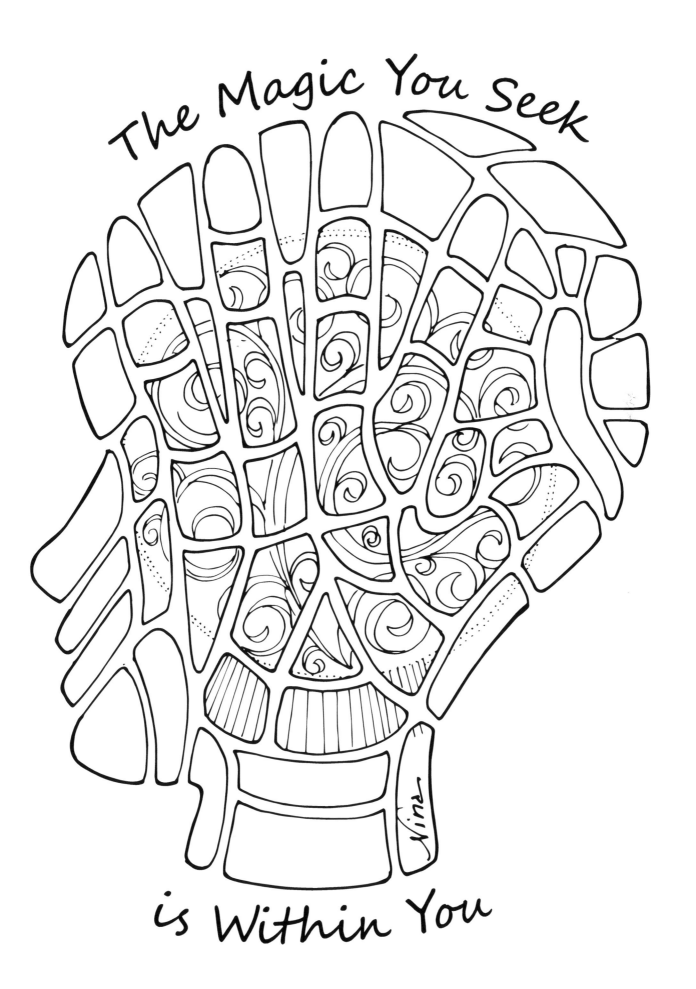

Just do you! Just be you! It sounds simple, but sometimes it can be difficult to figure out who or what you are. There are many voices telling us who we "should" be, and what we "should" think.

However, only you can know you! Only you have had your experiences. Only you know your likes and dislikes, your wants, your needs, your moods. Only you know your values, beliefs, priorities and habits. Only you know your passions, dreams and desires. Only you know your fears, strengths, weaknesses and limits.

Sometimes we get lost. We feel off balance or off center and it's easy to look outside ourselves to find who we are.

However, it's not outside, but inside we must look. You have all the expertise you need. Getting to know yourself is a powerful tool. It's the key to unlocking all that you are.

As you color, use the time as intentional "get to know YOU" time. Reconnect with yourself. Remind yourself of your dreams, your abilities, your strengths, your likes. Remind yourself who you are.

- *What are my likes and dislikes?*

- *What do I know to be true about me?*

- *What is truly important to me?*

- *What am I afraid of? What am I NOT afraid of?*

Take a moment to go deeper. Answer the questions below and record any musings, epiphanies, or thoughts you want to remember.

1. What are two strengths you know to be true about yourself?

_____

_____

2. What do you know about yourself that no one else knows?

_____

_____

"Don't you ever let a soul in the world tell you that you can't be exactly who you are."

~ Lady Gaga

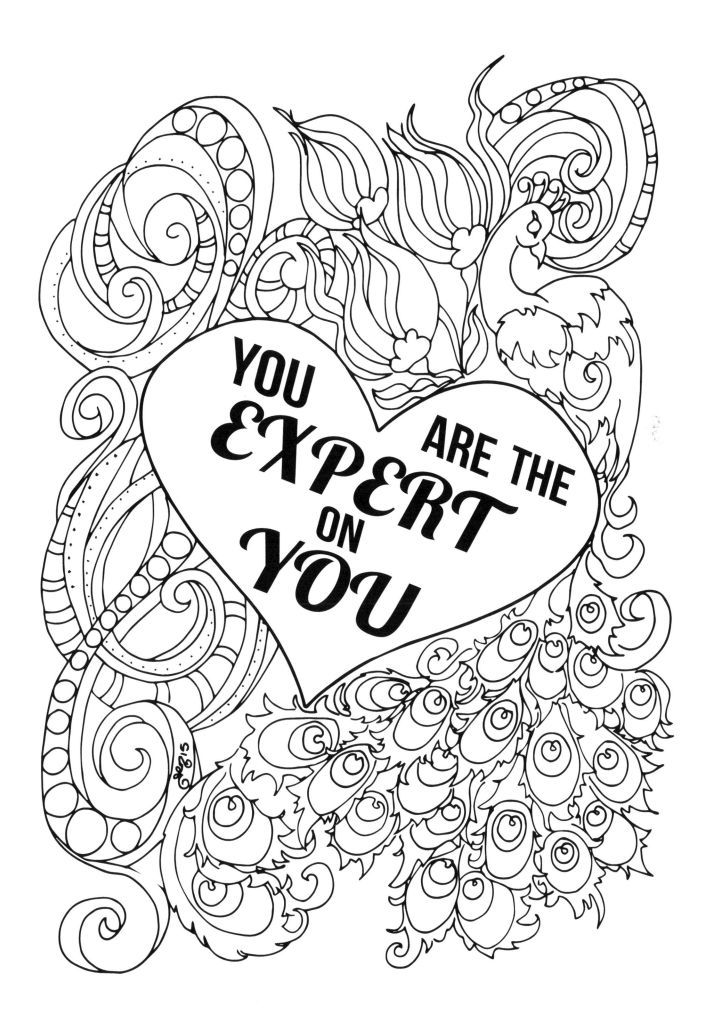

The world needs dreamers and creators, problem solvers and artists.

The world needs those who feel deeply, are honest and kind, compassionate and caring.

The world needs adventurers, wanderers, the unstoppably curious.

The world needs connectors, feelers, those who can't not care.

The world needs the bold ones, the unapologetically intense and focused.

The world needs the wild ones, the ones that won't be held back.

The world needs the quiet ones, who think and think and then think some more.

The world needs funny. It needs sad. It needs quirky and odd. It needs normal and boring.

You are the secret sauce. The world needs you to be you, to do what you believe in, to cultivate your unique talents and share them with us.

While you color, ponder just how unique you are and how that is exactly what the world needs.

- *What is uniquely you? That quality that only you can bring to life?*
- *What makes you come alive? What fills your spirit?*

Take a moment to go deeper. Answer the questions below and record any musings, epiphanies, or thoughts you want to remember.

1. What is one action you can take this week to feel alive?

_____

_____

2. Who is one person you can connect with this week that helps foster your unique self?

_____

_____

"Don't ask what the world needs. Ask what makes you come alive, and go do it. Because what the world needs is people who have come alive."

~ Howard Thurman

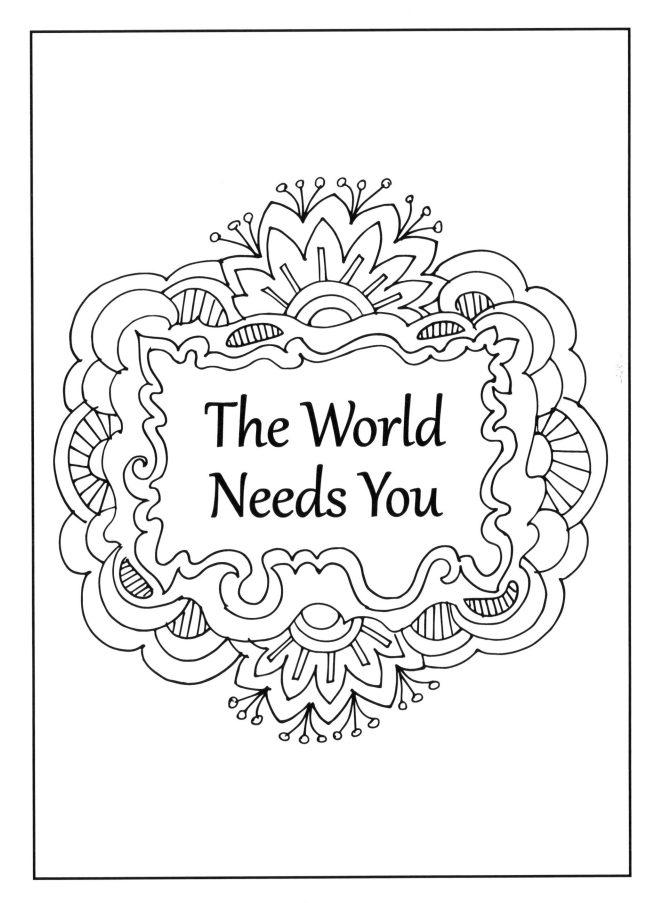

The World
Needs You

You are perfect. Exactly where you are. Doing exactly what you're doing.

With each day, each interaction, we learn. We learn what we like, and what we don't like. We learn what music excites us and which music makes us turn the channel. We learn that starting our term papers at 10pm the night before might not be the best way produce a well-written paper. Or maybe we don't (I still haven't learned this one).

When things don't work out it can feel like failure. But, although it can be heavy, the feeling of failure is not permanent. You explored, you experimented, you tried, and you learned what didn't work.

Think about how many times a baby, when learning to walk, stands up and falls back down. At what point does the baby say, "Well, that didn't work, I'm a failure, I give up." The baby doesn't. It just keeps trying, failing, trying again, and then trying again.

This is our portal to learning, to creativity, and to growth. It is our portal to progress.

While you color, take some time to think about what progress you have made in your life.

- *Where you were one month ago, one year ago, five years ago? What progress have you made?*

- *What do you know now that you didn't know last week? Last month?*

Take a moment to go deeper. Answer the questions below and record any musings, epiphanies, or thoughts you want to remember.

1. What is one thing that you have learned in the last week?

_____

_____

2. Write down a project that you're working on. What is one action you will take to progress on it this week?

_____

_____

"I'll try anything once, twice if I like it, three times to make sure."

~ Mae West

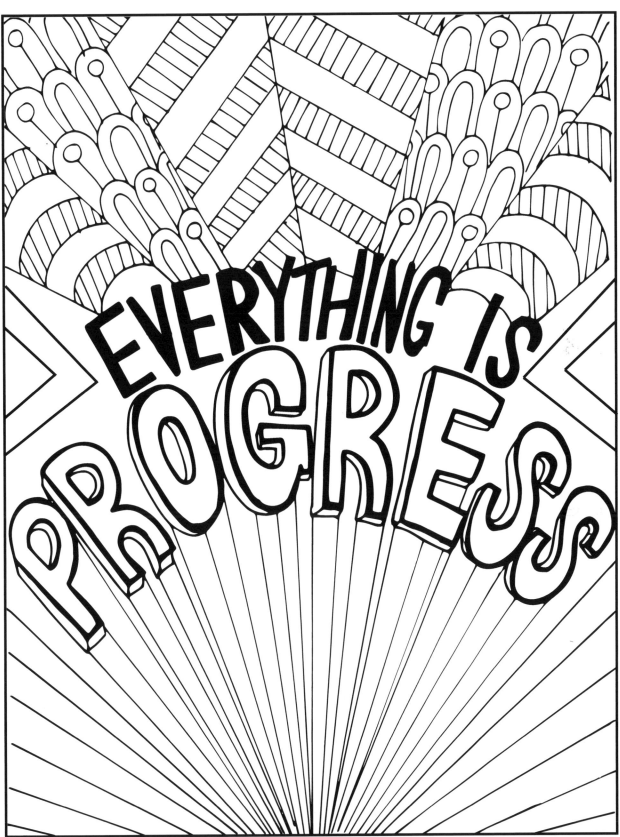

Where do your "shoulds" and "should nots" come from? There is a collective belief system that influences our lives. We learn it in school, as we interact with our friends, parents, and community, as we watch the news or the movies, and as we scroll through social media. There are entire industries that exist to influence and manipulate what we believe.

However, we have the power to CHOOSE what we believe. We have the power to question what we believe. When we become aware of our beliefs and explore them, we give ourselves power. What do you believe? Why do you believe and what could you do if you chose not to believe those limits?

Our beliefs determine what we manifest in life. What we believe becomes our reality.

While you color, focus on what you believe, what you know to be true, and be willing to explore where that comes from and why.

- *Explore your "shoulds" and "should nots."*
- *What do you know to be true about yourself and what you are capable of?*
- *What beliefs do you want to actively choose?*

Take a moment to go deeper. Answer the questions below and record any musings, epiphanies, or thoughts you want to remember.

1. What do you know to be true? Write down two things you choose to believe.

   a. I believe _____

   b. I believe _____

2. How will you pay attention to what you believe this week?

   _____

   _____

"You manifest what you believe,
not what you want."

~ Sonia Ricotti

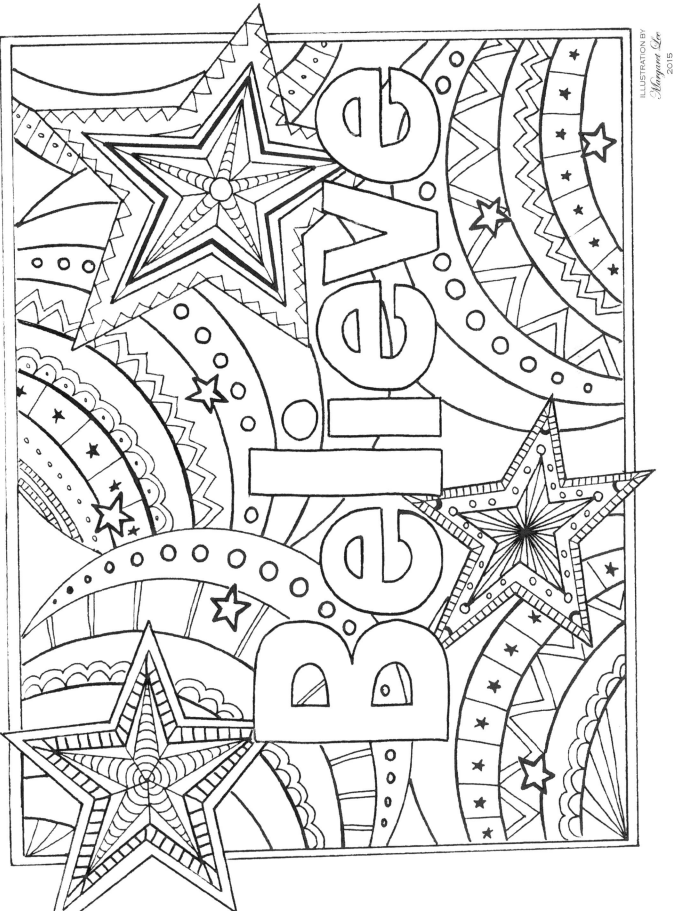

Abracadabra. Fairies and Unicorns. Elves and dwarves. Crystal Balls. Magical thinking.

Nope, we're not talking about that kind of magic.

Just like every fairytale begins with "Once upon a time," every morning you wake up and have the power to create the day, to invite magic into your day. Magic exists all around us. It's what happens when we notice the symphony in the chaos. It's in the everyday, regular things of life – and it's fascinating.

What is at the center of magic? IT'S YOU! You, fully aware of your power and doing all the things in your life that support you in being as wonderful as you are.

While you color, explore where you find the magic in life, what that feels like, where you find it, and how you can infuse your life with it.

- *When do you feel magic? What does it feel like?*
- *What is possible when you feel the magic?*
- *How do you spark your own magic?*

Take a moment to go deeper. Answer the questions below and record any musings, epiphanies, or thoughts you want to remember.

1. What is one of the experiences you remember that felt magical? What made it so?

_____

_____

2. What is something that you can do to spark magic in your life?

_____

_____

"Those who don't believe in magic will never find it."

~ Roald Dahl

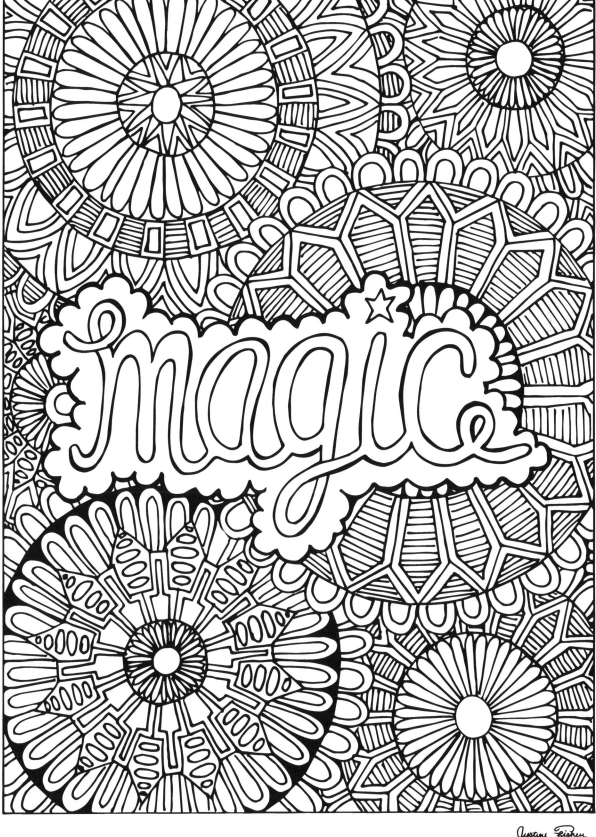

The world is deliciously complex.

Some of the best parts of life are those unexpected experiences, the ones we could never have planned for – that best friend you met on that train ride you weren't supposed to take, that favorite book you found at the garage sale your friend dragged you to, or that new idea you had talking to the person next to you at the baseball game.

Adventure, exploration, and discovery require searching for the answers to the questions you have while also allowing space for new questions to arise. Mystery is where inspiration finds us, where the unknown steps in and gives us new information.

Certainty or mystery? It's not a question of "either or" – It's a matter of "both, and."

Set your intention. Be purposeful in your thoughts and actions, but leave room for the mystery.

While you color, ponder how mystery plays a part in your life.

- *What things do you do that create space for mystery? Traveling? Reading? Exploring?*
- *What are the experiences you've had that have been unexpected and unplanned?*
- *What role does mystery play in your life?*

Take a moment to go deeper. Answer the questions below and record any musings, epiphanies, or thoughts you want to remember.

1. What is something in your life that happened because there was space for mystery?

_____

_____

"In the measurement world, you set a goal and strive for it. In the universe of possibility, you set the context and let life unfold."

~ Benjamin Zander

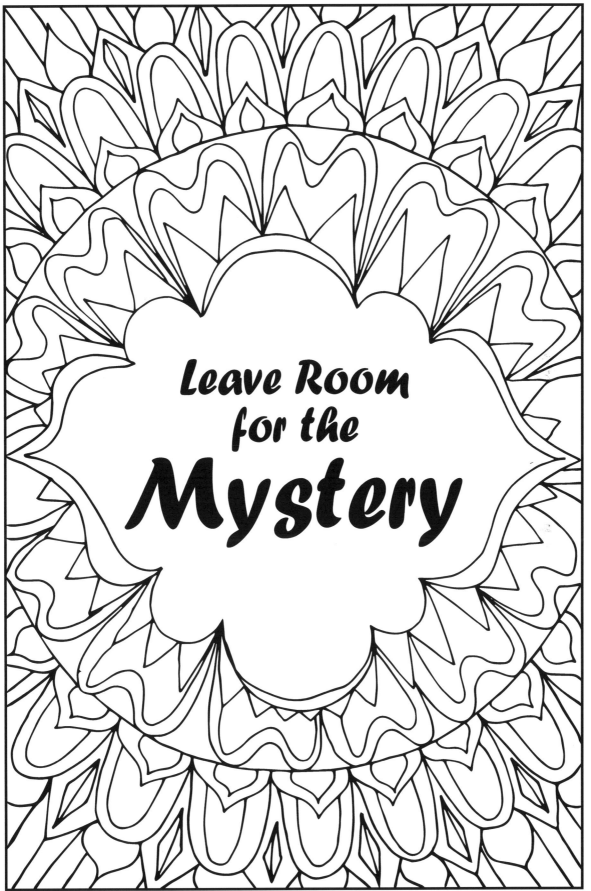

"Come on baby, light my fire," crooned Jim Morrison. But, the reality is that it's no one's job to keep your fire lit but you. Yup, that's right – YOU ARE IN CHARGE. You are responsible for keeping your fire lit – for keeping your heart charged at full capacity. Only you know those secret nooks and crannies of your heart, and what is needed to keep them aflame.

While you color, explore what you know about how to keep your fire lit and what reminds you what is possible when you keep your heart full.

- *What warms your heart? What lights you up?*

- *What changes when your heart is full? What are you capable of with a full heart?*

- *What are your "go to's" for recharging your heart? (e.g. listening to music, connecting with friends, watching TED talks, reading a good book, taking a walk outside, hitting the gym, etc.)*

Take a moment to go deeper. Answer the questions below and record any musings, epiphanies, or thoughts you want to remember.

1. What is one activity you will do this week that helps you "light" your fire?

_____

_____

2. Who is one person you will connect with this week that helps you recharge your heart?

_____

_____

"Go within every day and find the inner strength so that the world will not blow your candle out."
~ Katherine Dunham

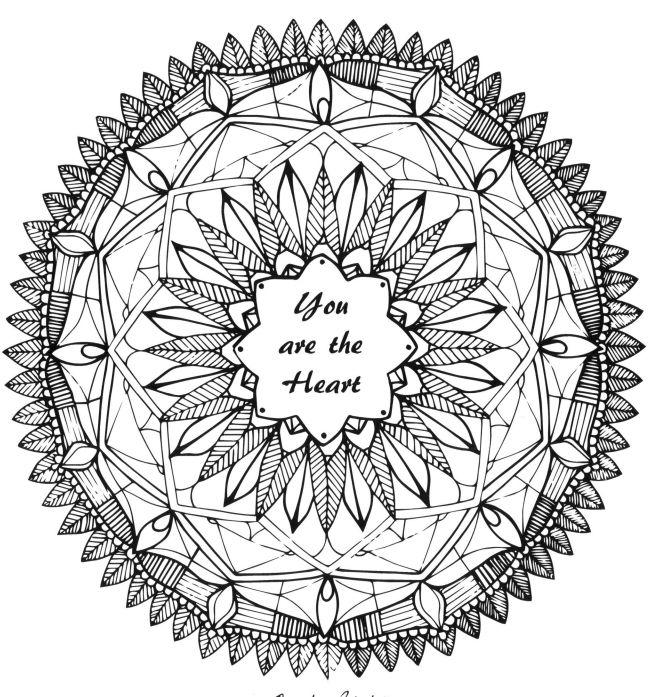

You
are the
Heart

"Put your own oxygen mask on first." Our capacity to support and care for others is directly related to our capacity to support and care for ourselves. Logic tells us that we must take care of ourselves first. However, in the practice of self-care, making space for others first is often the norm.

You, at the center, at full power, at full capacity, are what the world needs.

While you color, take a look at which beliefs have you helping others before yourself. Also, take a look at what self-care looks like for you (Is it a walk on the beach, listening to music, taking a dance class, or just doing those tasks you've been putting off?).

- *What more are you capable of when you are well cared for, rested, and centered?*

- *What does self-care look like for you? What are the things you do that relax and rejuvenate you, that relight your spark?*

- *What strategies do you have for supporting yourself and your self-care?*

Take a moment to go deeper. Answer the questions below and record any musings, epiphanies, or thoughts you want to remember.

1. What is one thing you will do this week to take care of yourself? What's your "oxygen mask" for the week, so to speak?

_____

_____

2. What are your favorite self-care rituals? How do you feel when you do these rituals?

_____

_____

"The greatest thing in the world is to know how to belong to oneself."

~ Michel de Montaigne

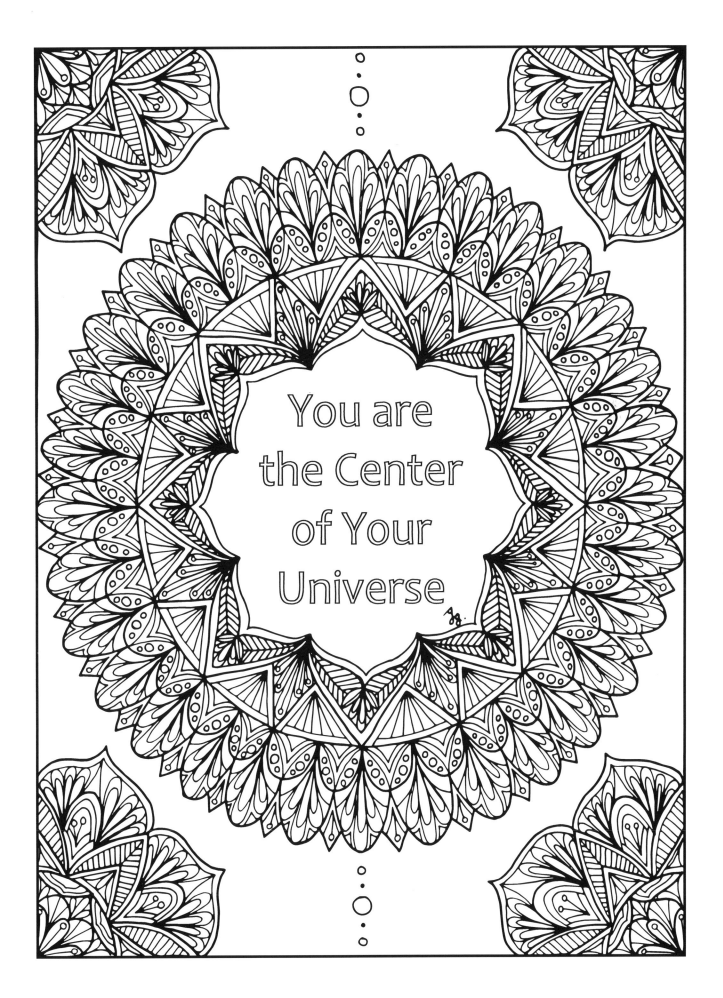

Life is a dynamic experience. It is an opportunity to learn, develop, and evolve into the biggest and best version of yourself. Emotions come and go. Experiences happen. Perceptions are altered. Personalities evolve. Our personal capacity expands.

When we expand our personal capacity, we are able to do and handle things that we couldn't before. We increase our knowledge of ourselves and our self-confidence. When we expand and grow into our full selves, we influence those around us to do the same.

Nurture your appetite for learning. Cultivate your ability to be comfortable with growth. Question your boundaries, try new things, and foster your creativity.

While you color, become aware of your personal abilities and cultivate your curiosity about learning and growth.

- *What are some of things that you want to learn about, that you can't wait to try?*

- *What does it feel like when you expand what you know?*

Take a moment to go deeper. Answer the questions below and record any musings, epiphanies, or thoughts you want to remember.

1. What is one thing that you can do now that you couldn't last year?

_____

_____

2. What is one area that you want to focus on expanding this year?

_____

_____

*"We must let go of the life we have planned, so as
to accept the one that is waiting for us."*
~ Joseph Campbell

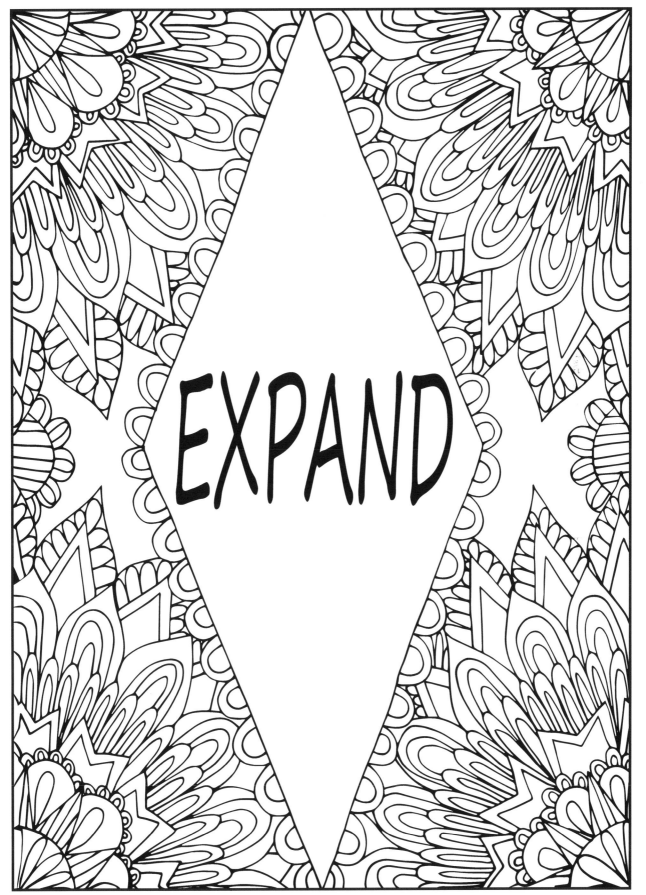

This is a call to action, to check your relationship with procrastination, to "get up and get busy" and to just do your "thang".

In today's fast-paced, digitally driven world, it's easy to get caught up in the overwhelm of being busy and at the same time feel like you're on the losing end of the procrastination battle.

This is a call to look inside at that thing you've been wanting to do, that you've been putting off, that you've been waiting for the perfect circumstances to begin.

This is a call to check in with yourself and what is important to you, to check in with those things that you care about most in the world and look to how you can contribute to making a difference in the world.

While you color, ponder what you think of when you hear this phrase.

- *What have you been waiting to do?*
- *What things would you like to do, if you only had the time?*
- *What are the reasons you put off starting? Why have you been putting them off?*

Take a moment to go deeper. Answer the questions below and record any musings, epiphanies, or thoughts you want to remember.

1. What is one thing you've been too busy to start?

_____

_____

2. What is one action you can take this week towards getting started on it?

_____

_____

3. What is one thing you've been putting off starting?

_____

_____

"One day you will wake up & there won't be any more time to do the things you've always wanted. Do it now."

~ Paolo Coelho

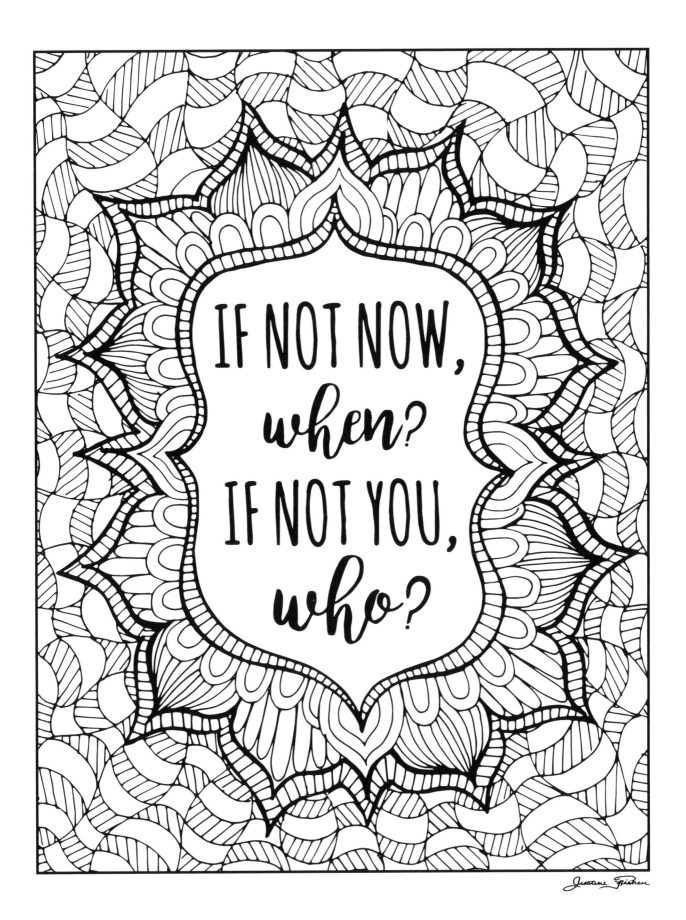

Life is short. We hear this repeatedly, but somehow its relevance slips away from us until something happens, an event that triggers us to remember, once again, how short life really is. Sadly, these triggering events never seem to be happy events – but instead seem to include some sort of significant loss.

However, You don't need to wait for a trigger, you can help yourself remember.

What are you waiting for? **HINT: It's Time. Today.**

Whose permission do you need? HINT: The only permission you need is your own.

While you color, turn your attention to TODAY! Be present with where you are at this moment and to check in with yourself about what you've been waiting for. What is that "thing" you've been putting off getting done, that phone call you keep forgetting to make, that project that you've been waiting for someone to give you "permission" to start.

- *What's on your waiting list?*
- *What are you waiting to get started on? How would it feel to get started on that?*
- *What is important to you that you want to make sure you do?*

Take a moment to go deeper. Answer the questions below and record any musings, epiphanies, or thoughts you want to remember.

1. What is one of the things on your "waiting" list?

_____

_____

2. What are two (small) steps you can make to get started?

_____

_____

"There is no future, there is no past. There's only us, There's only this. Forget Regret or life is yours to miss. No other road, no other way, No day but today."

~ RENT

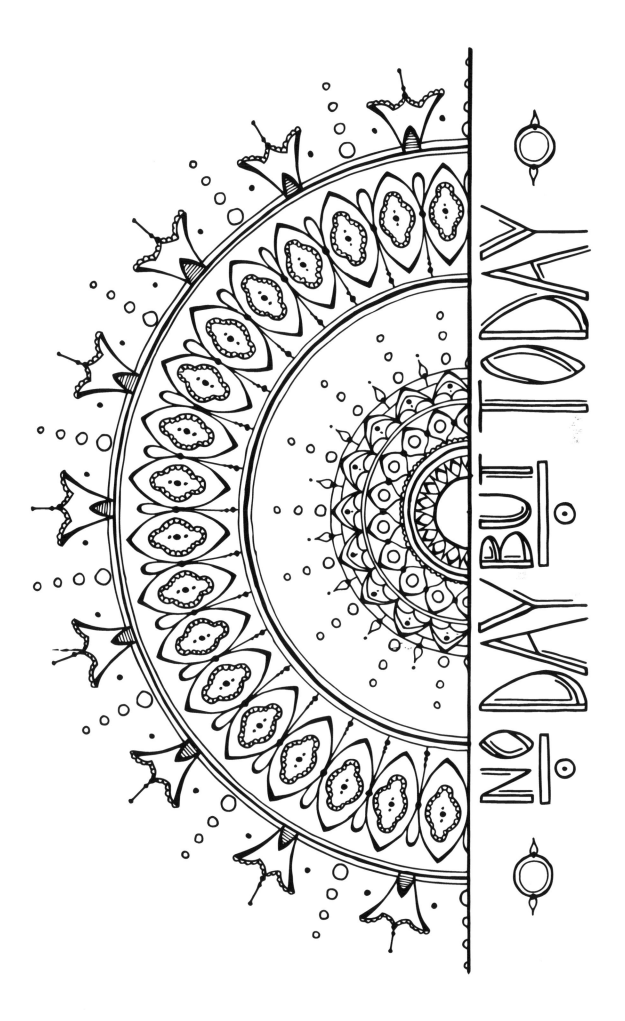

Your mission, should you choose to accept it, is to be possible!

YOU are possible. Everything you want in life is possible. You have the potential, the ability and the capability to be anything you want to be. And, you tap into that possibility by CHOOSING.

Yes, you get to CHOOSE who you become, by deciding, every moment, to become the "you" that you know you can be.

Will fear show up and try to scare you away from what you want? Oh yeah!

Will fear challenge you with expectations, the "shoulds" and "should nots?" Of course!

But your mission, should you choose to accept it, is to choose, every day, to be all that you have the potential to be.

While you color, explore everything you're capable of – not just what you've been told you can do, not just what you think "should" do.

- *What do you KNOW, in your heart, that you're capable of?*
- *What would be/is possible when you feel balanced, centered, and confident?*

Take a moment to go deeper. Answer the questions below and record any musings, epiphanies, or thoughts you want to remember.

1. Write down one thing you can do this week to help you feel balanced, centered, and confident.

_____

_____

2. What are two things that YOU know that YOU'RE capable of?

_____

_____

"Nothing is impossible, the word itself says 'I'm possible'!"

~ Audrey Hepburn

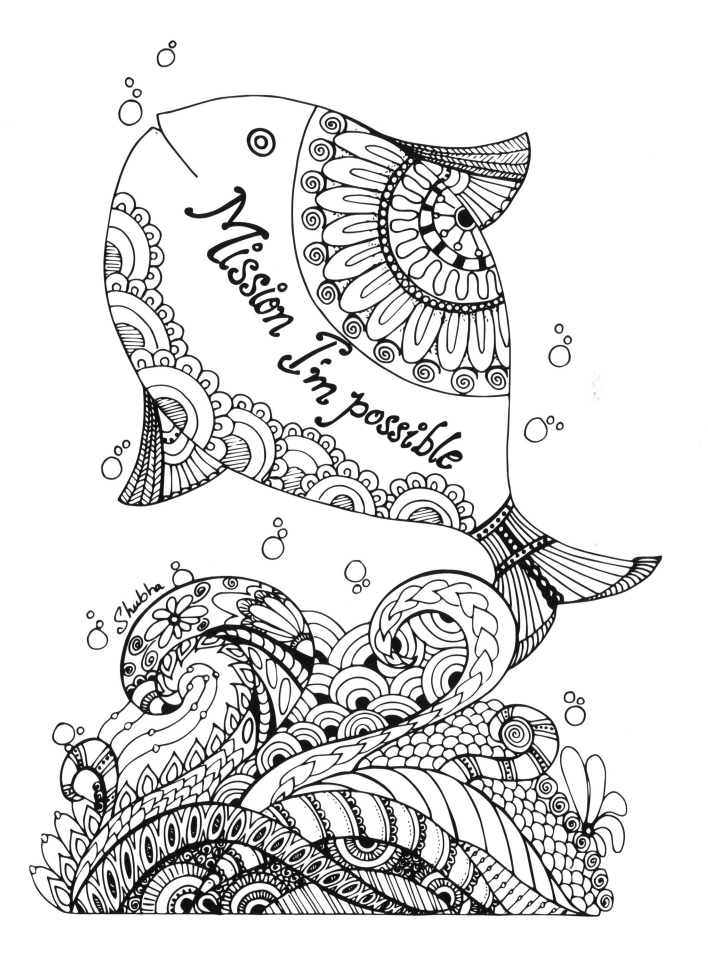

"Well, today's a good day, I woke up." This is always my 99 year old grandfathers response when I ask him, "How are you today?"

Gratitude, or the quality of being thankful, is an affirmation of the good things we've received in life. Gratitude is also a recognition that these things don't need to come from external sources. Rather, gratitude can be found everywhere – in the big things and, especially, in the small things.

Noticing what we are thankful for and practicing gratitude helps in experiencing positive emotions (joy, optimism, happiness, etc.). Gratitude can help us act more compassionate and generous, and can help us feel less lonely or isolated. Studies have shown that actively being aware of what we're grateful for has a positive effect on our immune system and blood pressure. Yes, you could even sleep better.

While you color, check in with yourself and what you are grateful for.

- *What are the things (big and small) you're grateful for in your life?*
- *How do you show that you are grateful for something?*
- *What does it feel like when you're grateful?*

Take a moment to go deeper. Answer the questions below and record any musings, epiphanies, or thoughts you want to remember.

1. What is one of the big things you are grateful for? Why are you grateful for it?

_____

_____

2. What is one of the small things you are grateful for? Why are you grateful for it?

_____

_____

3. What is one thing you'll do this week to express gratitude?

_____

_____

"Gratitude can transform common days into thanksgivings, turn routine jobs into joy, and change ordinary opportunities into blessings."
~ William Arthur Ward

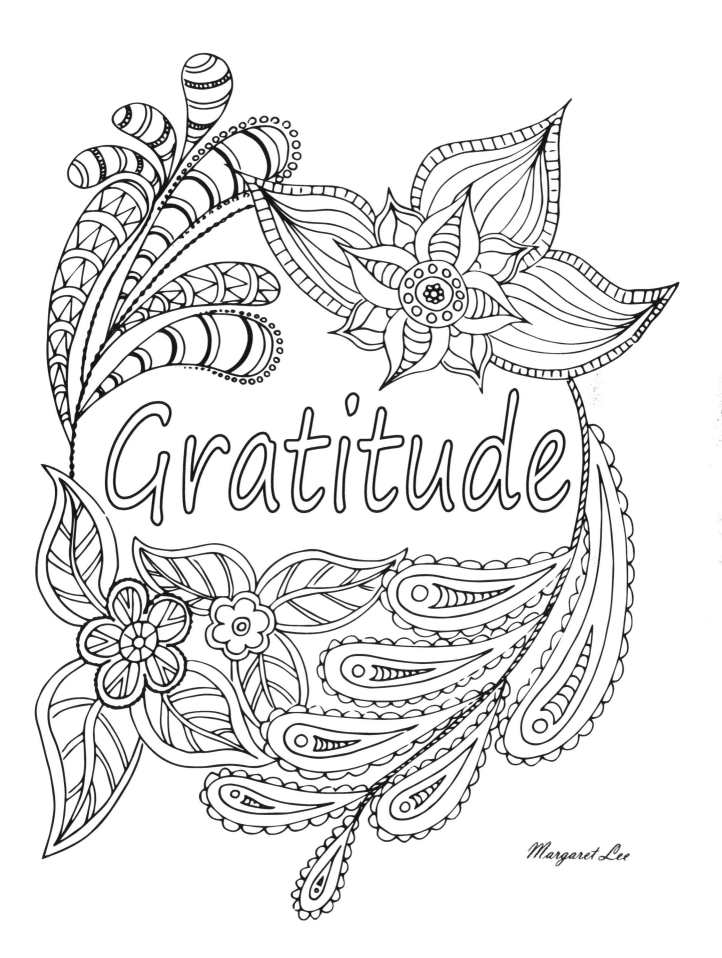

Any time we generate a new idea or thought – we are creative.

Creativity is not a "holy grail" only obtainable for those with talent. Every thought, story, thing you do is an act of creation.

To be creative is the ability to make new things, to think of new ideas, to use your imagination to come up with original ideas and innovative/different approaches to a task.

If you watch children – every child creates. If you put on music, they move. They don't worry about how to do it or whether they're "doing it right" – they just create movement.

We are ALL creative: A chef mixing ingredients, a teacher designing classroom activities, a CEO managing and running a company. What will you create?

While you color, explore your own creativity, identify where you are creative, and get to know the conditions that help stimulate your creativity.

- *What does 'being creative' mean to you?*

- *How are you creative?*

- *When are you most creative? What conditions foster your creativity? What do you need to do to fire up that creative spark – music, place, clean, dirty, outside, inside?*

Take a moment to go deeper. Answer the questions below and record any musings, epiphanies, or thoughts you want to remember.

1. What are your conditions for creativity? Place, music, people, time of day?

_____

_____

2. What is one thing you will do this week to spark creativity?

_____

_____

*"I am my own experiment.
I am my own work of art."*

~ Madonna

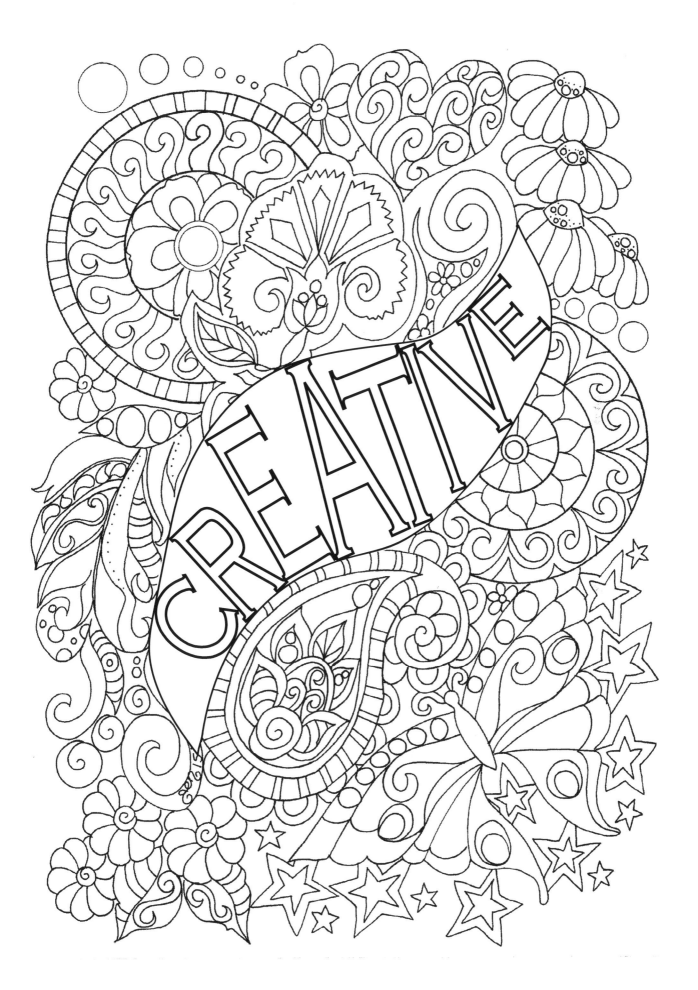

"Make it so." – Captain Picard.

Those things in your life that you wish existed, those things that you keep hoping will appear – it is up to you to create them.

We have the capacity to create our lives, to direct them. We are the architects, the pilots, the writers, and the choreographers of our own lives.

There is only one person responsible for what you create in your life. That person is you. With our actions, we create. With our actions, we change ourselves. With our actions, we change the world.

While you color, get in touch with what you want to create in life.

- *What ideas do you want to bring to life?*

- *Who are the people creating things in this world that you admire most? What qualities do they possess that contribute to their creativity?*

Take a moment to go deeper. Answer the questions below and record any musings, epiphanies, or thoughts you want to remember.

1. What is one idea you have that, if brought to life, would change your world?

_____

_____

2. What one step can you take this week to create one of these ideas?

_____

_____

"Everything you want is out there waiting for you to ask. Everything you want also wants you. But you have to take action to get it."

~ Jules Renard

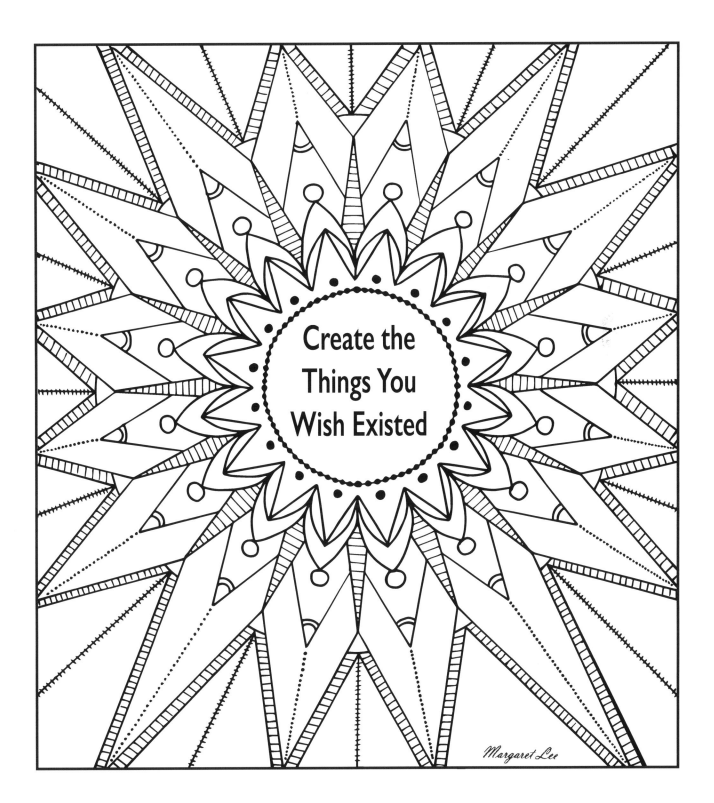

Create the
Things You
Wish Existed

Margaret Lee

This is it. Today is the day. Take that first step. Now.

We delay. We wait to start. The reasons not to start are easy – the conditions aren't quite right, something is missing, someone's permission is needed, there's not enough time to complete the task in one shot, etc. The "if onlys" and the "shoulds" keep us from starting, they keep us from doing the things that we want in life.

Take one step, even if it's a baby step. It creates momentum. And momentum begets more momentum.

Seize the day. Carpe Diem. Pick each day as if it were a ripe fruit.

Now is that moment you've been waiting for. Not tomorrow. Not next week. Not next year. Now.

While you color, think about what how good it feels to complete something, to start and to finish.

- *What would it feel like to get "that" project started?*
- *What are your "if onlys" and your "shoulds?" What are they keeping you from?*

Take a moment to go deeper. Answer the questions below and record any musings, epiphanies, or thoughts you want to remember.

1. What was the last project you started and completed?

2. What is one project that you've been putting off? What is one small step you can take towards it this week?

"There are seven days in the week and someday isn't one of them."

~ Wayne Dyer

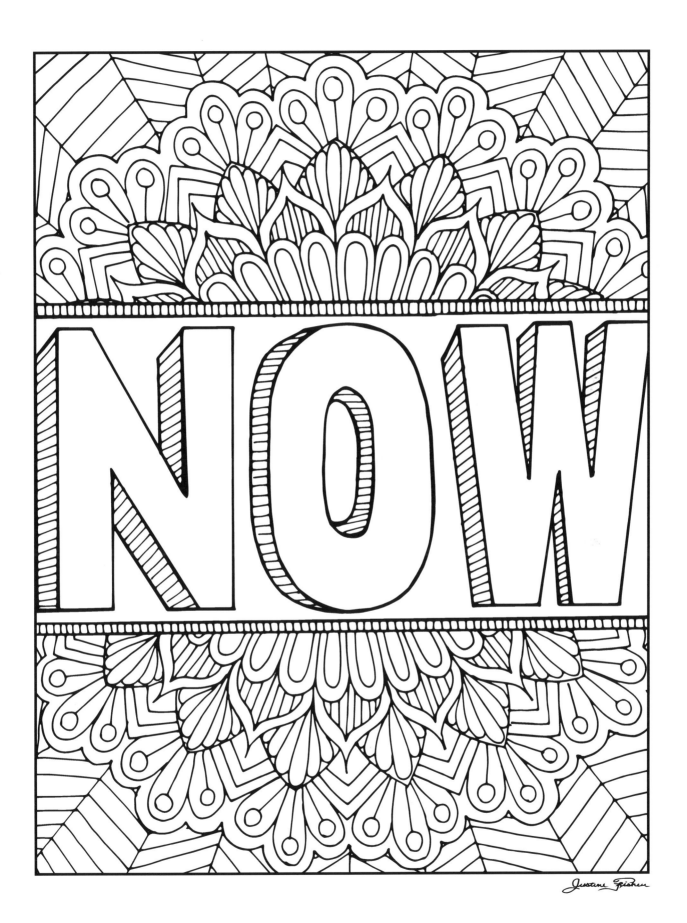

"If you can dream it, you can do it." – Walt Disney

The way we think about ourselves, our "mindset" according to Carol Dwek, guides how we see possibility. Often we develop a way of thinking, a routine we are comfortable with. And, the more comfortable we are, the harder to challenge or break from the routine.

Possibility emerges from cultivating a "growth mindset" – or a way of thinking that believes that our abilities are not fixed, but can grow and develop. It is possible to cultivate your mindset and cultivate possibility by feeding your curiosity and fueling the desire for learning. Dive into a book, have deep conversations with new people, follow a rabbit hole researching a topic on the Internet.

New people, new ideas, new adventures, and new connections await you.

Those possibilities are always there, waiting for you to choose them.

While you color, ponder your curiosities, what makes you need to know more.

- *What topics excite you and fill you with curiosity? What do you just need to know more about?*
- *What's on your bucket list? What are those things that want to do... someday?*

Take a moment to go deeper. Answer the questions below and record any musings, epiphanies, or thoughts you want to remember.

1. What is one item on your bucket list?

_____

_____

2. What is one action you can take this week towards this item?

_____

_____

"When you get to a place where you understand that love and belonging, your worthiness, is a birthright and not something you have to earn, anything is possible."

~ Brené Brown

All
Things
Are
Possible

Intention without action does not create change. It is only through action that change occurs.

Taking the step to do something, to move your idea into action, is where most of us get stuck. This is where the "what ifs" come in, where self-doubt takes us for a ride, and where getting stuck with "I don't know the right first step" happens.

Sometimes we make plans to make plans. Sometimes we think things through to the 'N'th degree. Sometimes we get distracted by the next big, shiny, bright idea. Squirrel!

It's time. Do what you need to do. The world needs you to take the next step forward to create what only you can create.

Inspiration & Intention + Action = Change & Transformation

While you color, explore your ideas and your inspirations and look for that next step.

- *What's on your "to do" list? What are those things that have been lingering, waiting for you to start moving forward?*

- *If you did that ONE thing, what else would be possible as a result?*

Take a moment to go deeper. Answer the questions below and record any musings, epiphanies, or thoughts you want to remember.

1. What are three SMALL things on your TO DO list?

_____

_____

2. What is one BIG thing on your TO DO list?

_____

_____

3. What is one SMALL thing that you will take action on this week?

_____

_____

"Vision without action is merely a dream. Action without vision just passes the time. Vision with action can change the world."

~ Joel A. Barker

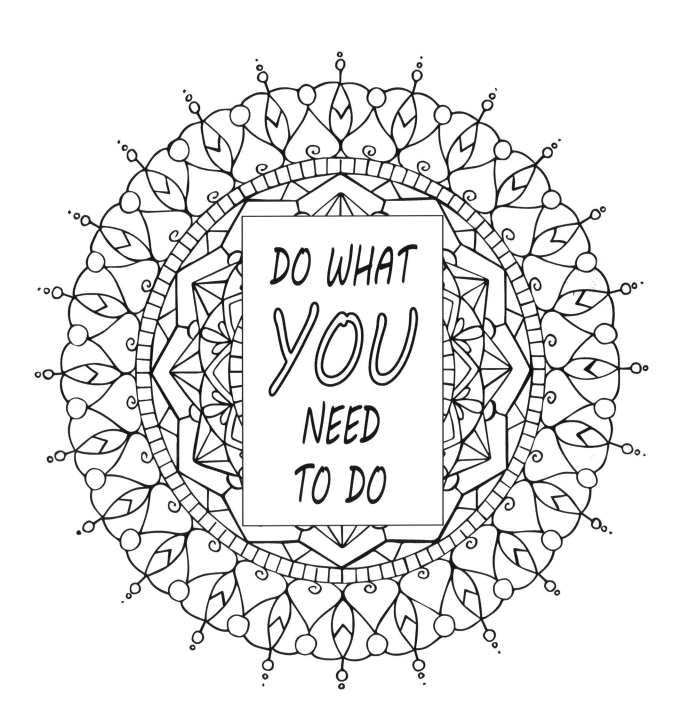

In Japanese, "Nana-Korobi, Ya-Oki." In English, "Try try again."

Edward Scissor Hands, BeetleJuice, Nightmare Before Christmas. Tim Burton's list of successful movies goes on. In an interview about his success – Burton was quick to mention that for every successful movie there are a couple hundred movies he's made that no one has seen.

Michael Jordan has shared similar sentiments, "I've missed more than 9000 shots in my career. I've lost almost 300 games. 26 times, I've been trusted to take the game winning shot and missed. I've failed over and over and over again in my life. And that is why I succeed."

Many of us are glad that Mark Zuckerberg "tried" to start a social network. And the environment is benefitting from Elon Musk's repeated attempts, and eventual success, at building an electric car.

It doesn't matter that you didn't succeed, but rather, that you tried. It doesn't matter that you fell, only that you get back up and try again.

While you color, connect to your own resilience and ability to persevere.

- *What keeps you going when you want to quit?*

- *What things can you do now because you had to keep trying?*

Take a moment to go deeper. Answer the questions below and record any musings, epiphanies, or thoughts you want to remember.

1. What is one skill you have now that required repeated attempts?

_____

_____

2. Who is one person you know that encourages you to keep trying?

_____

_____

"The only source of knowledge is experience."
~ Albert Einstein

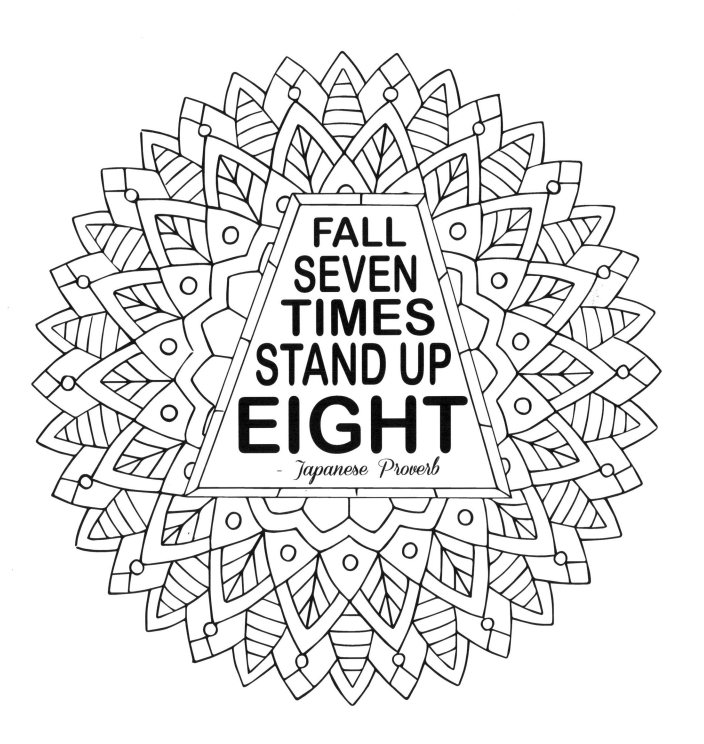

From the Latin word inspirare, or to breathe life into something, inspiration can feel magical and mythical – those moments of transcendence, when time disappears and your senses are amplified. Inspiration knows no class, race, or gender – it is a beautiful gift that each one of us can access.

Finding inspiration is good for you. It creates focus, fills you with a sense of purpose and can move you towards your goals. It awakens you to new possibilities and allows us to transcend our limitations as we create new pathways to achievement.

Although we'd like to control inspiration, that isn't always the case. But, we can work to create conditions that increase the chance of inspiration activation – which include, making space and time for inspiration, aligning ourselves with what is important to us, and being open to new experiences.

While you color, connect with your inner compass and check in with where you find inspiration.

- *Where do you find inspiration? Is it in music, in certain places, or when you do certain things?*

- *What does being inspired feel like in your body? Is it light? Is it pulsing energy? Is it tingly?*

- *What are the places and people who inspire you?*

Take a moment to go deeper. Answer the questions below and record any musings, epiphanies, or thoughts you want to remember.

1. What are three things that inspire you? (music, locations, poetry, conversations, books, etc.)

_____

_____

2. What one thing can you do this week to light your inspiration fire?

_____

_____

"True inspiration overrides all fears. When you are inspired, you enter a trance state and can accomplish things that you may never have felt capable of doing."

~ Bernie Siegel

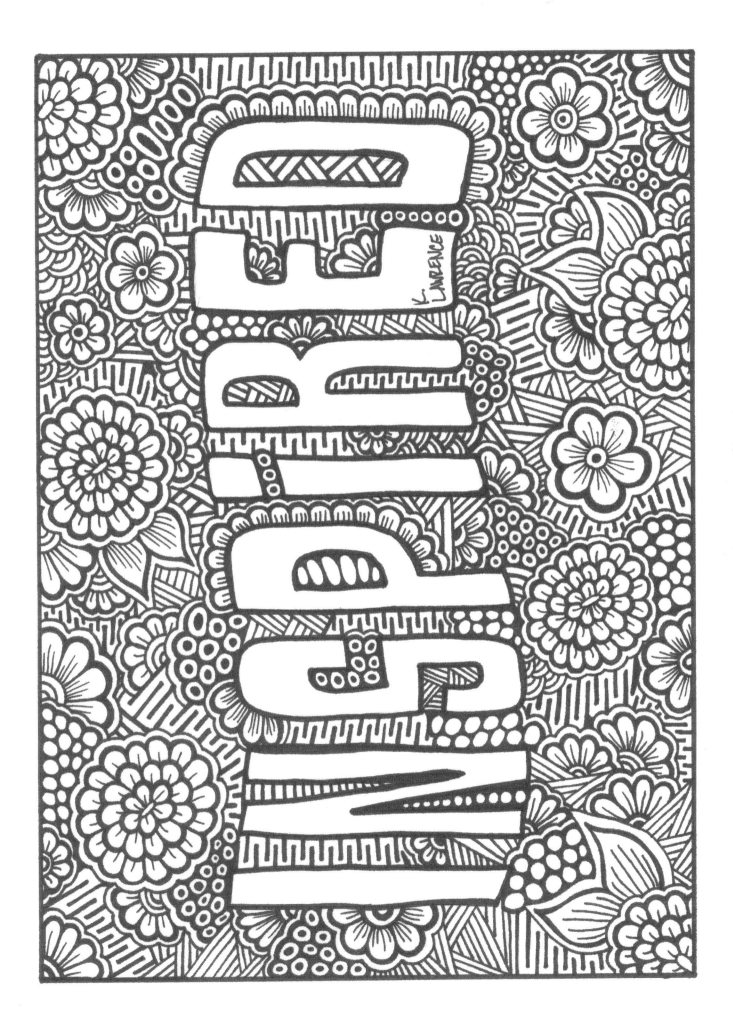

There is nothing more powerful than recognizing that you have the power to create your world, to create your reality.

Your power resides in how you talk to yourself, in the story you create about what you are capable of.

Your power comes from knowing yourself, knowing who you are, and being yourself.

Your power resides within you. Your power is ready and waiting for you to define it and own it.

It is being unapologetically you. It's about pursuing becoming who you are fully.

You are a force of nature.

While you color, get in touch with what it feels like when you feel powerful. Whether it's physical strength or emotional strength, think about what power feels like for you.

- *What does being powerful mean to you?*
- *Where do you draw your power come from?*
- *What is possible for you when you feel powerful and strong?*

Take a moment to go deeper. Answer the questions below and record any musings, epiphanies, or thoughts you want to remember.

1. Who are the people that you consider powerful? What qualities do they represent?

_____

_____

2. What do you do to develop your own strength, your power?

_____

_____

"When you catch a glimpse of your potential, that's when passion is born."

~ Zig Ziglar

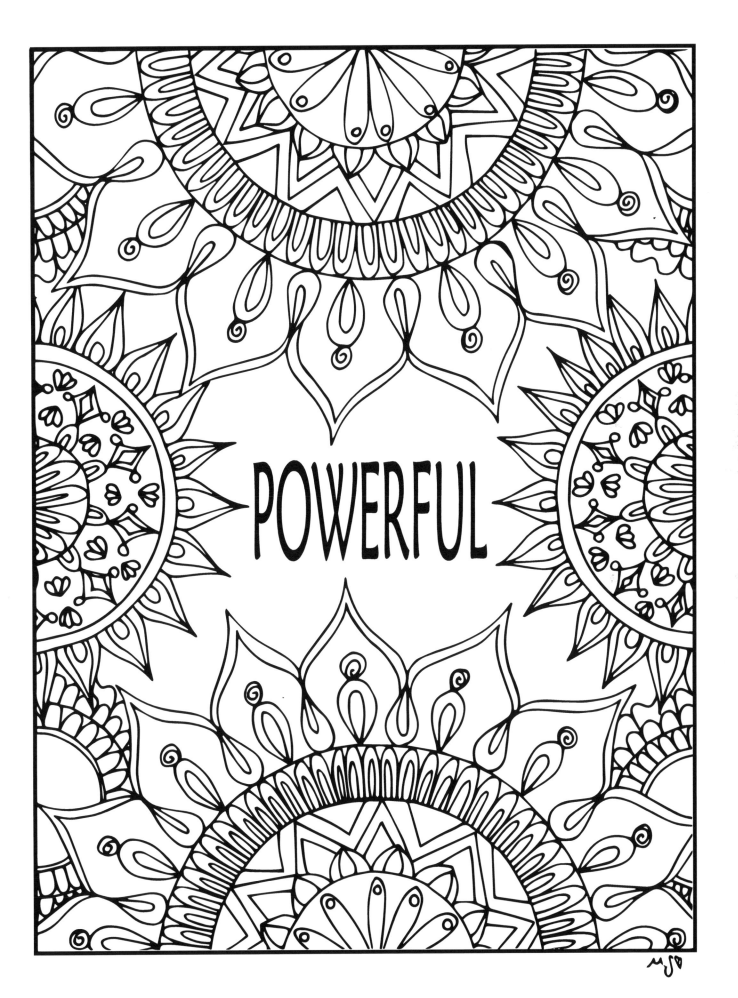

It's Electric, Boogie Woogie Woogie - The Electric Slide.

You know it when you feel it. Spirited. Vital. Animated. Passionate. Brilliant. That exhilarating feeling of energy and enthusiasm, that effervescent joy that makes you want to sing and dance and jump about to music!

This feeling can be generated externally – going to your favorite concert, a promotion, a great vacation, a night out with friends.

This feeling can also be generated internally – working on your sense of balance, meditating, identifying your purpose.

While you color, explore what helps you feel vibrant and identify how you can purposefully tap into and nurture it.

- *How do you feel when you are feeling vibrant? What are some words that describe that feeling for you?*

- *What are the things you know will help you "get your groove" on to feel vibrant?*

- *What shifts about you when you feel vibrant?*

- *When you are feeling vibrant, what else is possible?*

Take a moment to go deeper. Answer the questions below and record any musings, epiphanies, or thoughts you want to remember.

1. What's your "go to," "I just gotta feel vibrant right now" place? (turn up the music, take a drive, a walk in the woods, etc.)

_____

_____

2. Write down one thing you'll do this week to feel vibrant.

_____

_____

*"Sometimes your joy is the source of
your smile, but sometimes your smile
can be the source of your joy."*

~ Thich Nhat Hanh

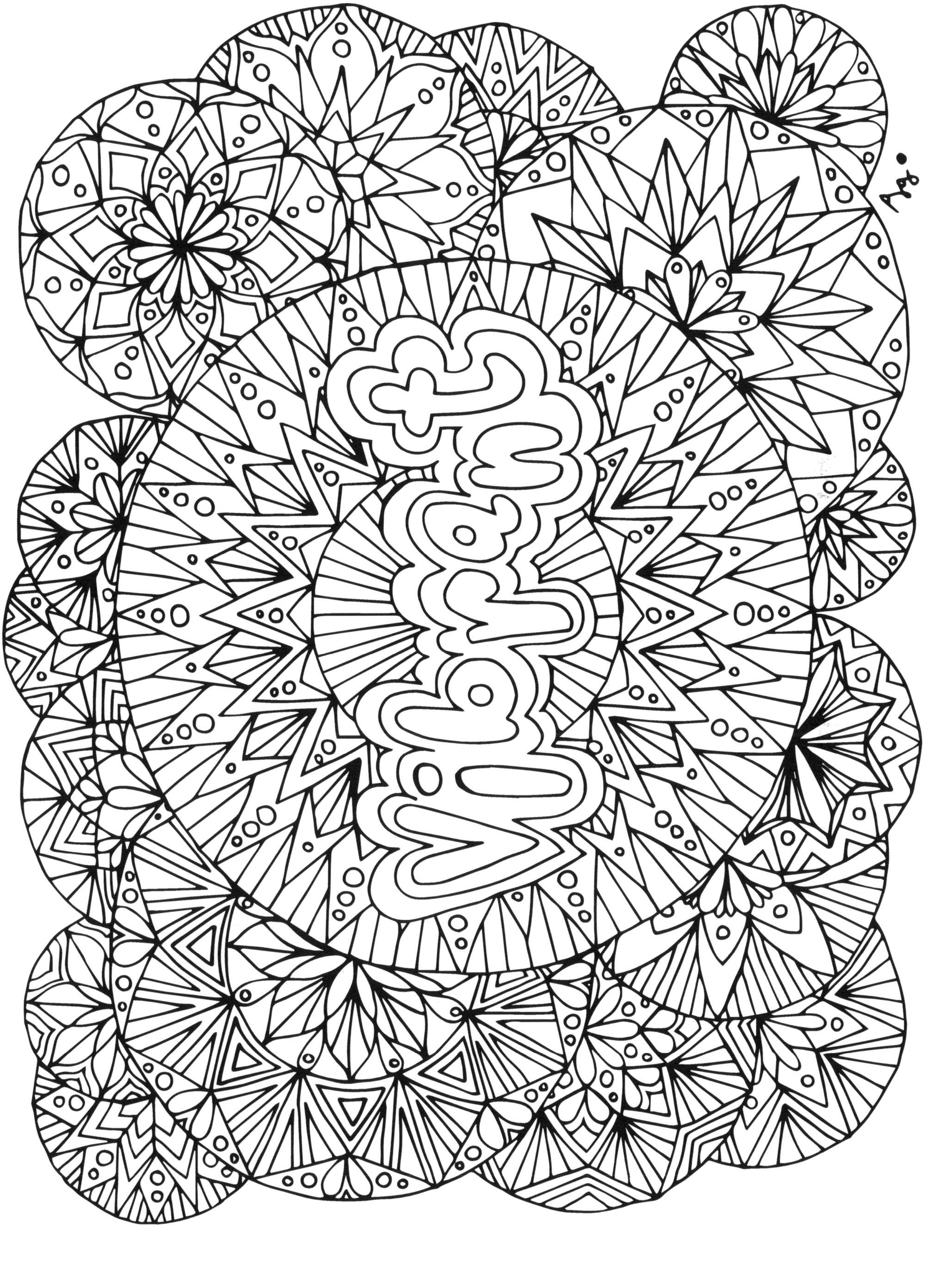
vibrant

Choosing is our right and our privilege.

To choose to be happy, to be content, to be confident.

To choose to strive, to be inspired, to find your purpose.

To choose what affects you and how it affects you.

To choose your attitude and your reaction.

To choose to hope, to reach out, to encourage and understand.

To choose to act or to choose to stand still.

With every choice, with each action, you have the power to decide who YOU are each and every day.

Regardless of the choices you made yesterday, last week, last year, today is a new day. What will you choose today?

While you color, think about what choice means to you.

- *Make a mental list of the things you get to choose? What are the small choices you have? What are the big choices you have?*

- *If you could choose anything, and you can, what would you choose?*

Take a moment to go deeper. Answer the questions below and record any musings, epiphanies, or thoughts you want to remember.

1. What is a choice you made in the past that you are proud of?

_____

_____

"Our lives are a sum total of the choices we have made."

~ Wayne Dyer

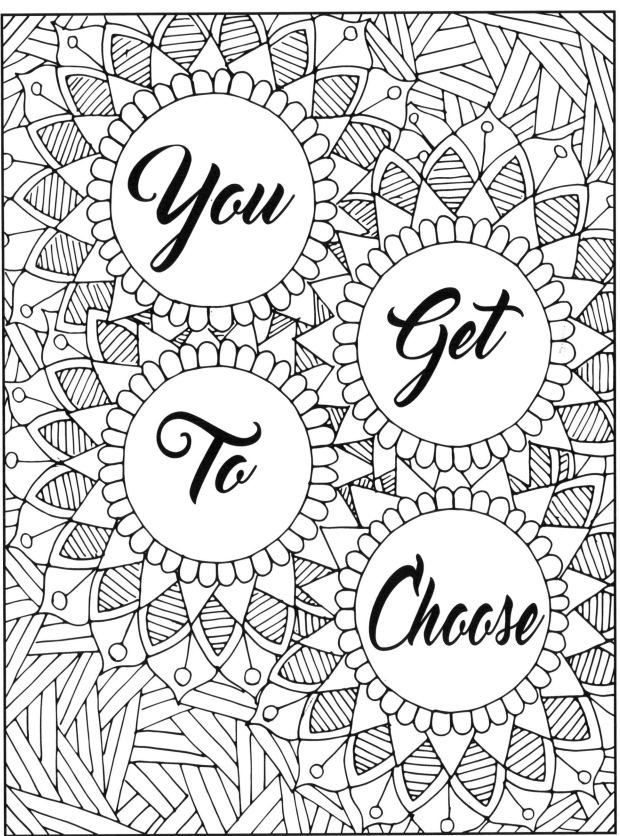

LOVE is more than the romantic, "I love you" that movies and pop music talk about. Love is complex. Love is sophisticated. Love is diverse. Love is healing. Love is alive. Love is something we all experience in its different forms.

There are many types of love.

EROS: Romantic, passionate love.

PHILLIA: Friendship, companionship, chosen love.

STORGE: Familial love, parental, unconditional love.

AGAPE: Humanistic, altruistic love.

LUDUS: Flirtatious, playful love.

PRAGMA: Practical, long standing love.

PHILAUTIA: Self-esteem and self-love.

We all experience love in each of these areas. Fostering each type of love can increase your overall capacity for love and relationship.

While you color, think about the different types of love you have in your life and your own definition of what love is.

- *Where do you find love in your life? What kinds of love light you up?*

- *Who are some of the people that inspire love in you?*

Take a moment to go deeper. Answer the questions below and record any musings, epiphanies, or thoughts you want to remember.

1.   What are the types of love that are present in your life?

_____

_____

2.   What is one action you can take to develop love, whatever type, this week.

_____

Piglet: *"How do you spell 'love'?"*
Pooh: *"You don't spell it, you feel it."*

~ Winnie the Pooh

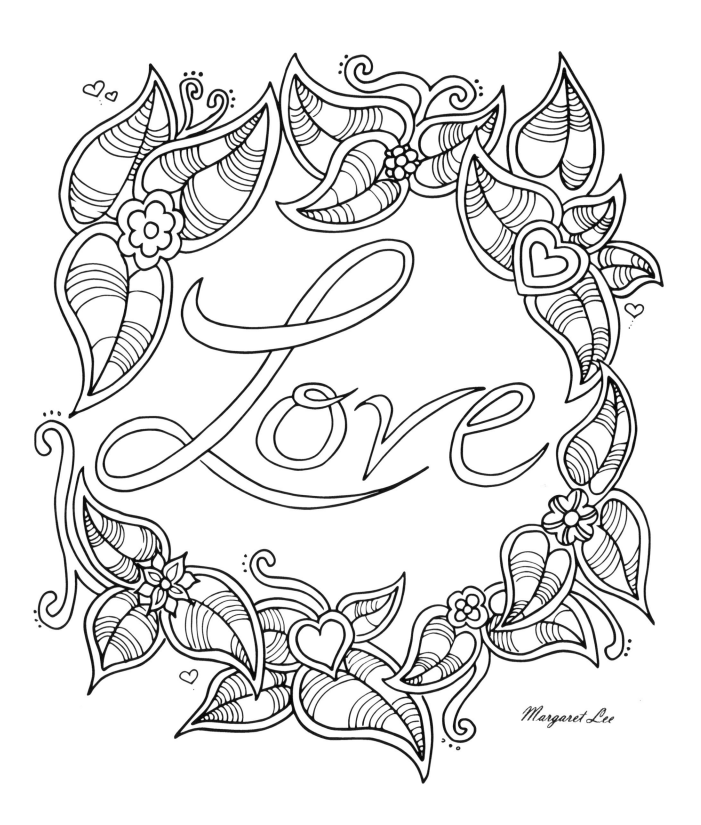

Margaret Lee

That driving force. That call you must answer. That connection to something that you feel at your core.

No one but YOU can know what your purpose is.

Don't fret if you haven't found yours. Finding purpose takes finding yourself. It takes getting to know you and what is most important to you.

It can be a connection to something larger, it can be a contribution to something you care about, it can be just unleashing that inner part of yourself that can't be restrained any longer. It could be saving the world, righting wrongs, challenging social norms, traveling to every country on the planet.

Whatever it is, YOU get to choose. Your purpose is what YOU say it is.

While you color, take time to explore your purpose – whether you've found it already or are still looking.

- *What is your purpose?*
- *What are you drawn to? What makes you feel the most alive?*

Take a moment to go deeper. Answer the questions below and record any musings, epiphanies, or thoughts you want to remember.

1. What does your perfect day look like – from the moment you jump out of bed to the moment your eyes close at the end of the day?

_____

_____

2. What is one thing you can do this week to explore your purpose?

_____

_____

*"It is in your moments of decision
that your destiny is shaped."*

~ Tony Robbins

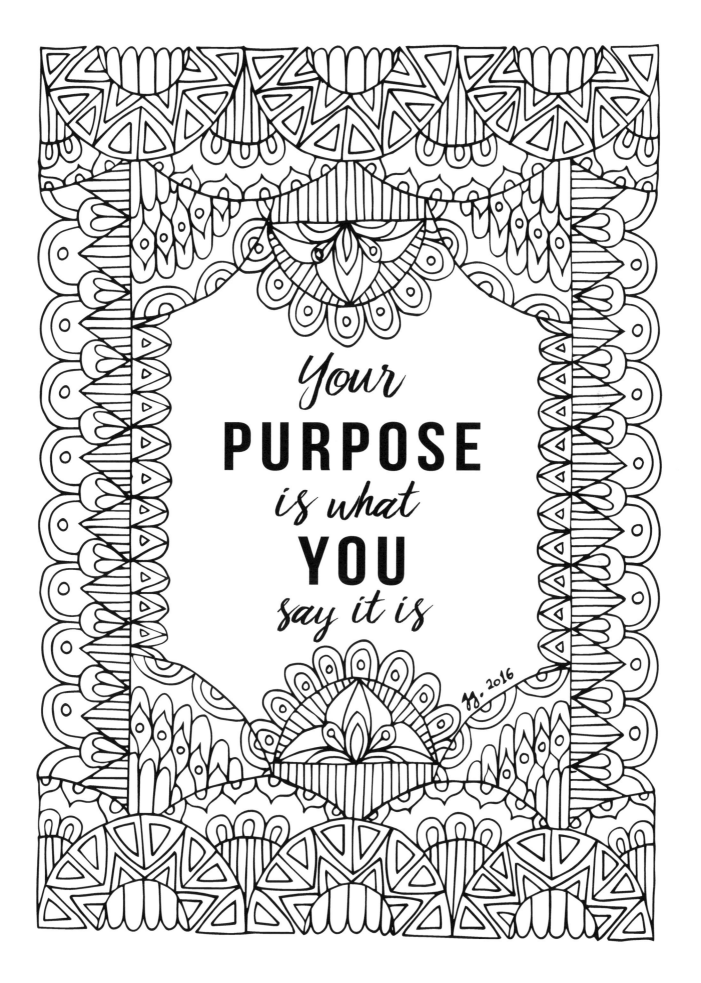

Happiness is not a pursuit. It is not something to aspire to or to obtain. It does not depend on having something before it can be felt.

Happiness is within us. It is our true self. It is our center, our light, our joy, our laughter and our freedom. It is our kindness, our affection, our love, and our caring. It is appreciation and gratitude. It is the source of our possibility.

Happiness is abundant. And, as we cultivate happiness, it expands. It has no limit.

While you color, get in touch with the happiness inside yourself.

- *Where does happiness come from for you? Is it family, friends, career, music, art?*
- *What things help you amplify your happiness?*
- *When you feel happy, what is possible?*

Take a moment to go deeper. Answer the questions below and record any musings, epiphanies, or thoughts you want to remember.

1. What are your favorite ways to generate happiness?

_____

_____

2. What is one thing you can do this week to generate happiness?

_____

_____

"Always find time for the things that make you feel happy to be alive."
~ Don Miguel Ruiz, Jr - The Mastery of Self

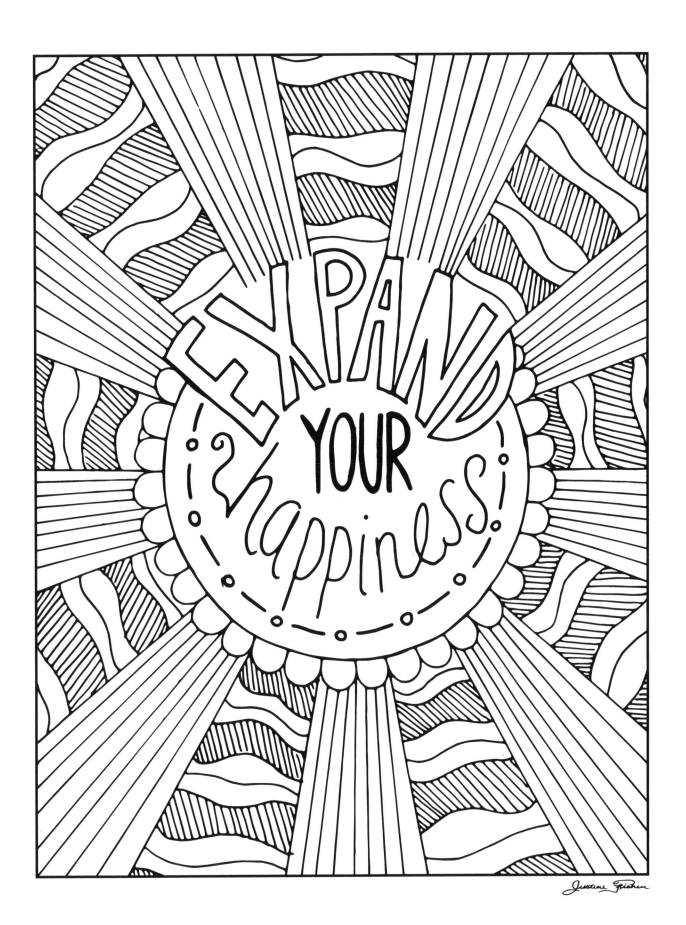

"To Thine Own Self Be True." - Shakespeare

Bravery means different things to different people and in different situations.

It can mean fighting the fight until the very end or it can mean knowing when to wave the white flag. It can mean speaking up and standing out, or it can mean choosing to remain silent.

Bravery can mean taking risks, being the only one who believes, not knowing what the "right answer" is and doing it anyway. Bravery can also mean being content with what is.

What bravery means is personal. It is specific and unique to you. Bravery comes from that quiet voice inside of you, the one that is aligned with your inner compass. It is not a matter of ignoring your feelings and never being afraid. Rather the opposite, bravery emerges from knowing yourself and honoring what you know to be true.

While you color, explore what it means to be brave.

- *What do you think of when you hear the word brave?*
- *What does it mean to you to be truly brave?*
- *What are your most treasured moments of bravery?*

Take a moment to go deeper. Answer the questions below and record any musings, epiphanies, or thoughts you want to remember.

1. Describe what bravery means to you.

_____

_____

2. What is one brave thing you've done, that you didn't think was brave at the time?

_____

_____

*"You are braver than you believe, stronger
than you seem, smarter than you think,
and loved more than you know."*
~ A.A. Milne, Winnie the Pooh

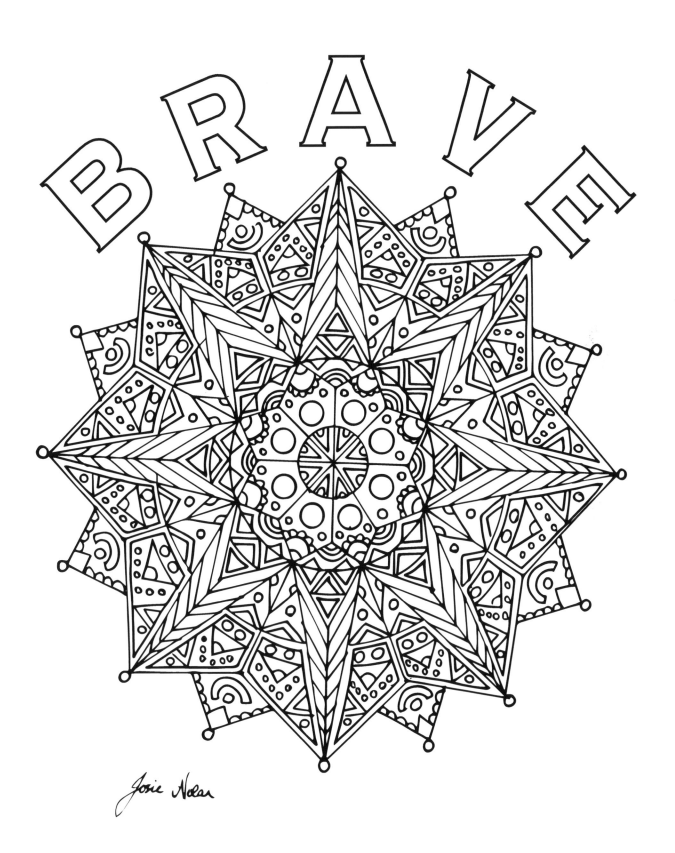

ABOUT THE COLORING PROJECT™ & ANDREA KOEHLER

The Power of Positive Coloring blends the benefits of coloring with guided mindfulness exercises. Developed by Andrea Koehler, her work with coloring is influenced by her Training & Development work with Fortune 500 companies. Coloring as a path to mindfulness has been described as a "trip to the mental gym accompanied by a mental massage."

Andrea founded The Coloring Project™, as a way to harness coloring's meditative mental drift and use it as a tool for transformation and self-discovery. Her work is used in corporate and non-profit leadership events, team building exercises and community engagement events.

Andrea currently resides in Seattle – when she's not dancing (Salsa, Bachata and Afro-Brazilian, even Zumba), you can find her at the theatre watching Musicals.

THE ILLUSTRATORS

AUSTRALIA
Jenni Dee Mills
Josie Nolan

CANADA
Justine Fisher
Margaret Lee

INDONESIA
Nadira Maharani Ramses

SINGAPORE
Shubha Balasubramanya

THE UNITED KINGDOM
Leonnie Spencer
Phoebe Sutteclif

THE UNITED STATES
Kristin Lawrence
Madison Scott
Magda Petrou
Michael Seidel
Nina Scott

Visit www.TheColoringProject.com to learn more about The Coloring Project, our mission and our featured artists. You can also find us on all the "socials."

ACKNOWLEDGEMENTS

About 10 years ago, a set of circumstances triggered my awareness that I was not where, or who, I wanted to be. My own journey of self-discovery and of learning about how much I got in my own way had been set in motion. A long and winding road followed. And now – I am here – blending my love of self-discovery with the creativity of coloring.

That journey was not a solo one. Along that road were amazing people and connections, without whom I would not be exactly where I am now.

To **Tamir,** for being with and loving all of me, for holding me accountable to show up and be ALL of me, for coaching as a form of compassion even when I don't want it, and for more laughs than I can recount.

To **the Parentals** and familial relations, thank you for living your creativity – each in your own right – through mad crocheting skills, through dance and movement, through cars and design, and through hair coloring skillz that defy comprehension.

To **my crew,** ALL the people in my life who continue to light my fire, thank you for hours on the phone talking about everything and nothing, for always hatching plans to better the universe and for being there with me when I can't be there for myself.

To all the **authors and thinkers** (Don Miguel Ruiz & family, Danielle LaPorte, Wayne Dyer, Stephen Covey, Paolo Coelho, Brené Brown, Daniel Goleman, Malcolm Gladwell, Angela Duckworth, Mihaly Csikszentmihalyi, ad infinitum), whose words and ideas give me fertile ground from which to grow.

To my **soul sisters** - Catie, Karen, Cecile, Susan, Pats, and Jennifer. To the **Impact Hub Seattle** for providing my "happy place" to create and for being a womb of support. A bow to **Myrcurial** and **Jackie** who have been supportive in ways they aren't even aware of. A toast to **Mr. Rivas** – I've got my CEO pants on now. To the entrepreneurial communities that support when I don't know what I don't know! To every one of the meetup members who agreed that an evening spent coloring and conversing was an evening well spent. To Made For Success Publishing, thank you for being open to a coloring books and supportive of projects extend farther than I can think about!

And a final thank you to YOU, the reader & colorer, who picked this book up, who thought hey – coloring and self-discovery – that sounds like a good idea. Thank you for sharing part of your journey with me.

"Alone we can do so little;
together we can do so much."

~ Helen Keller

P.O. Box 1775
Issaquah, WA 98027

www.madeforsuccesspublishing.com

First Edition: January 2017

Library of Congress Cataloging-in-Publication Data

Koehler , Andrea Reyna

The Power of Positive Coloring:
Creating Digital Downtime for Self-Discovery/Andrea Reyna Koehler

ISBN: 978-1-61339-822-7
LCCN: 201691471

Printed in the United States of America